HOW TO BE
SOBER
AND KEEP YOUR
FRIENDS

Flic Everett

PHOTOGRAPHY BY KIM LIGHTBODY

Hardie Grant

QUADRILLE

Contents

Introduction

There are plenty of great words associated with drinking: fun, sparkling, tipsy, giddy, crazy, wild, laughter. But when it comes to 'sober', according to the dictionary, we're suddenly looking at: serious, sensible, solemn, grave, sombre, severe and earnest. It seems there's a stark choice – you can either be fun, a massive laugh and have a great time with people who love hanging out with you over a bottle or three. Or you can be your old headmistress with toothache.

We are bombarded with messages that alcohol is the fast route out of Dullsville to a life of glitter and popularity, where mishaps become memories and a hangover is a small price to pay for friendship and fun. From adverts to greetings cards to social media, the idea is constantly hammered home that drink is our special reward for getting through the day. Whether it's prosecco o'clock fridge magnets, weary parents posting GIFs of housewives slugging gin or images of sun-dappled meadows with friends sharing cider and good times, there is no escape from the idea that booze is the answer to every ill.

I notice all this because I felt that way too. I loved alcohol like my own sister for decades. The worst it ever did to me was the occasional revoltingly painful hangover, usually forgotten by the next day, and some questionable kissing choices in my youth. I never hit rock bottom, I never answered a shame-faced 'yes' on any of those grim questionnaires about how much you're ruining your life by boozing (I mean, obviously I was late for work due to drinking the night before, sometimes, but who isn't?), I never suffered any booze-related injuries (unless you count once cutting my gum on some cocktail ice) and I can't think of any relationships that were dramatically harmed by my drinking. Some were probably improved.

So for years I staggered merrily along with my after-work glass of wine or three, and my out-for-drinks gin, and my 'may as well get another bottle' suggestions; as I bobbed through life supported by a gently flowing current of booze.

Then I got a bit older and suddenly, after a few glasses, I started to wake up feeling as though somebody had clamped my head in a vice, and stuffed a rotting guinea pig into my mouth while I slept. There was also the issue of The Flush – where one glass of wine would ensure a glowing red stripe across my face, like a menopausal badger. Eventually, I realised I was no longer really enjoying drinking, so I read a book about quitting, googled some tips and tried a week without a drink. That wasn't too hard, so I extended it… and felt much better. Waking up feeling normal was a huge bonus. Not having to worry about running out of wine was another. The only issue, in fact, was having to explain to people why I wasn't drinking as, 'No, I'm not an alcoholic – I'm just having a break from booze' is exactly what alcoholics would say, and I didn't want to start rumours that I was days from rehab.

So I had to think about all the other reasons why I was better off without booze. Once I'd done that, it was time to confront what was stopping me simply not drinking. Then I had to look at what might make me want to drink again… whether that was friends, social pressure, emotional states (and I have many) or just habit. And now I've done it – and I can tell you exactly how I managed it. A word of reassurance first: it's not nearly as hard as you think it's going to be.

Why Should I Quit?

There is plenty of information out there on why not drinking alcohol – or cutting down significantly – makes us healthier, happier people. The trouble is, we either don't want to hear it or don't believe it – or both. But the arguments are compelling, once you're prepared to put down the giant glass of pinot and, brace yourself, actually absorb them, instead of sticking your fingers in your ears shouting 'lalalalalala'. Such as...

*More energy

Ethanol is a poison. So when your exhausted body is spending the morning / entire day / whole weekend trying to purge the toxins from your bloodstream, there isn't much perky motivational energy left over. It also ruins your sleep – you may fall asleep faster, but you are more likely to wake up during the night and fail to get properly restorative REM sleep.

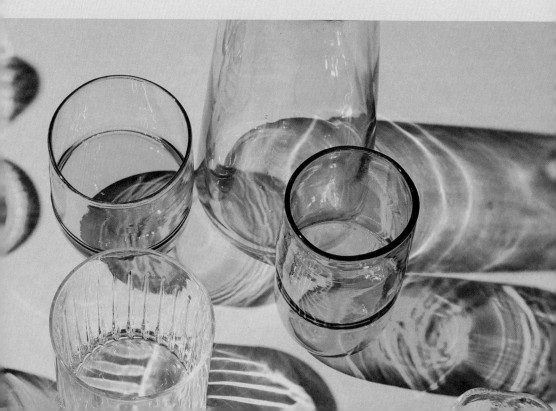

*Better skin

Alcohol is a diuretic, which means it makes you wee more and drains the water out of your cells – so dry skin and lines are far more obvious after a drinking session. It also causes inflammation, which manifests as redness and 'puffy face'.

*More money

I didn't want to work out even roughly what I used to spend on booze per month, let alone over an adult lifetime. But it was clear within a few weeks that there was magically more money in my account. I didn't have that little wince in the supermarket when the bottles clinked to a halt and the cashier said the total out loud. And eating out was instantly affordable, in a way it had never been before. The first time I opened a wineless restaurant bill, I thought it was a mistake.

*Less worry

As a fairly anxious person, I was very familiar with the whole heart-pounding scenario of waking at 4am and spooling through an evening of mortifying errors and terrible decisions. When you throw in 'stupid things I did and said while drunk', the resulting review could last for hours. Without booze, I only had to worry about the things I did sober.

*Better decisions

The trouble is, you have every intention of making good choices, and until the second drink hits your bloodstream, you're on track. You're going home after two drinks. You're not going home with your work crush. You're going to the gym first thing. You're not going to end the evening on the late bus with a reeking kebab in your lap. And it's all true, until the alcohol subtly loosens your resolve. Because you're having fun! Life is about enjoyment! Time is short! Until the regret and the hangover and the lost phone and keys (and possibly job and relationship) kick in. Without the drink, you know how much fun you're actually having. With it, it's horribly easy to mistake 'out of control' for 'having a great night'.

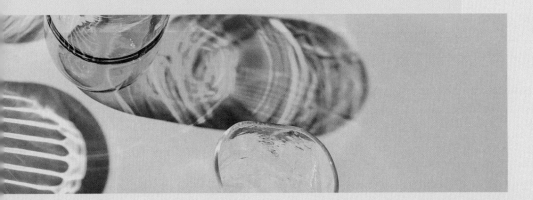

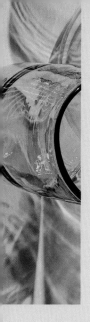

*Better health

The boring but valid one. Drinkaware recommends no more than 14 units a week for both men and women – that's six glasses of 13% ABV wine, or six pints of 4% ABV beer. Several recent studies have now found that there is no 'safe' amount of alcohol – it's better for health not to drink at all. And regularly drinking over the recommended limit or binge drinking (which means six or more units for women or eight or more for men in a single session – and no, going to the loo in between doesn't count) can contribute to heart disease, some cancers, liver disease, high blood pressure, stomach ulcers, depression, anxiety and, of course, some of the most crippling hangovers known to man. (I'm thinking particularly of the one when the cat purring on the bed sounds like a monster truck revving outside.) The government's advice is now that consuming any alcohol at all can be harmful.

*Better relationships

It's fair to say that, like most drugs, alcohol amplifies emotions. And if you're feeling a bit emotional anyway, it will take those normal feelings and blow them up into vast, unmanageable frenzies of hysterical passion. This is probably why I always had a taxi row with my ex after a night out, and why it hurts so much more when the person you fancy leaves the bar with someone else. It hurts mildly anyway, but on booze, it feels like the end of *The Notebook* crossed with *Titanic*. And you're much more likely to text your emotions as they happen to the last person you should be texting at 2am…

The problem
with explaining

//

Clearly, there's a ton of benefits to giving up – but if it were
that easy, everyone would do it. The biggest problem with
giving up drink, then, is not that you'll never have fun again,
or you'll suddenly become less attractive, or you won't know
what to do with yourself (we'll tackle all these points later).
The first big issue for many of us is, 'How will I explain this
to my friends?'

We tend to want to blend in with the crowd, no matter what
age we are – a reversion to the days when anyone separate
from the tribe would get speared, or eaten, or both. Or
maybe it's simply a throwback to the school bus, living in
fear of somehow standing out and having our bags thrown
round the upper deck. Either way, we tend to choose friends
because they are similar to ourselves, support our choices
and like us for who we are. Which is why, in a group of
people who enjoy cracking open a bottle or six, or downing
several beers at the bar, or whose social life is oiled by
an easy flow of G&Ts at the kitchen table, you suddenly
becoming a sober outlier is very difficult for everyone to
cope with. Because…

/ They feel like you're judging them.

/ You're holding up a mirror to their own drinking habits, and nobody likes that.

/ The group or friendship has always relied on certain traditions – meeting in the local, getting drunk together, encouraging each other to drink more – and now you're spoiling it.

/ Your shorthand and chats always involve booze: 'Can't wait for that glass of wine!' 'Let's meet for a well-deserved drink.' 'I'm putting the kids to bed, then pouring a massive G&T.' 'Cocktails for Helen's birthday – hope you can make it.' 'Beer after work?'

/ They worry you'll find them dull if you're not drinking.

/ They worry they'll find you dull if you're not drinking.

/ It's a bit like having a sober David Attenborough crouching in the bushes, watching the funny animals engage in their weird rituals. If you break out of the norm, you become the observer – and nobody wants to be observed when they're getting enjoyably hammered.

But… it is possible to cut down (or give up altogether) without feeling you're missing out on fun – and without losing friends. You'll just be leaving behind something that doesn't make you feel happy – and you won't turn into a preachy monster. Unless you want to, of course.

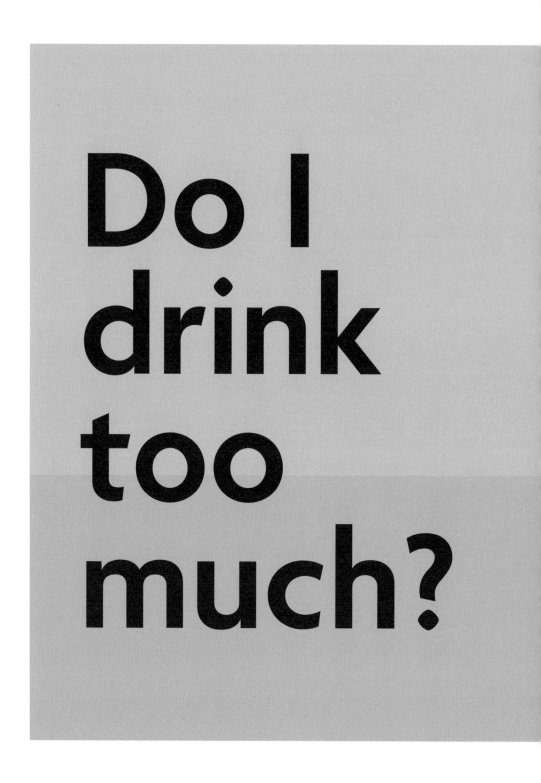

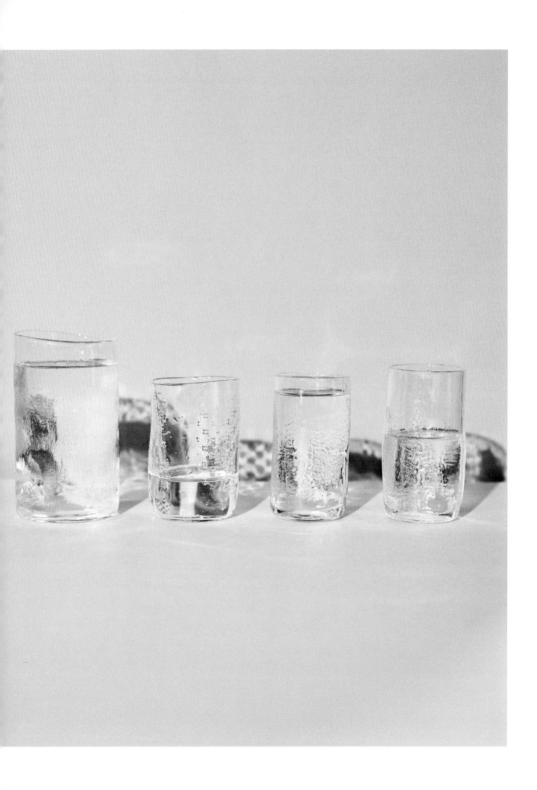

If you read government advice (and who doesn't, right?), any alcoholic drink is a bad drink – or 'a sad choice' as some teachers now say to wayward pupils. And if you are struggling to manage your drinking, it makes complete sense to cut it out altogether. Note I don't say 'try to' – you either drink or you don't. If you know that the first glass leaves you craving more, you're drinking because you're unhappy and you can't face life sober, or you're drinking to quell anxiety, to ignore the problems in your life or to cope with depression, things will not improve if you carry on drinking. Equally, if drinking affects your personality – makes you angry, violent, sad, gives you blackouts so you can't recall how you got home, makes you abandon your friends to wander home along unlit canals or enables other risky behaviours like sleeping with strangers or taking drugs, when normally you wouldn't dream of doing such things – well, you should probably consider cutting it out and see if life is easier to navigate.

Or perhaps you're just aware that you're drinking a bit too much; you don't want to quit, but equally, you definitely feel you should cut down. One (or several) too many hangovers that feel like the aftermath of a botched kidnapping, a good dose of 3am heart-pounding flashbacks and nauseated

~~~~~~

regret, the fallout from decisions you certainly wouldn't
make sober or simply a general, fuzzy awareness that you
could have more energy, enthusiasm and a lot more money
in your account if you didn't mindlessly open a bottle every
night… those are all good reasons if not to quit entirely, then
to cut down significantly.

If you're not sure – and let's be frank, most of us live in
a state of foggy denial about our drinking, basing what's
normal on our friends' average consumption, how much
our brother drank once (and he was fine!), the idea that
official statistics are guilt-tripping nonsense and the theory
that a little of what you fancy does you good – it's time to
cut through the denial and the 'I read an article that said
that red wine is good for you; pretty sure they said a bottle
a day?' arguments, and find out whether you really are
drinking too much, and more importantly why.

Because until you know what's motivating your drinking,
it's far, far harder to cut down or stop. So take the quiz, and
find out what's behind your boozing.

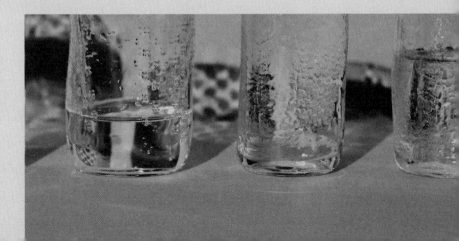

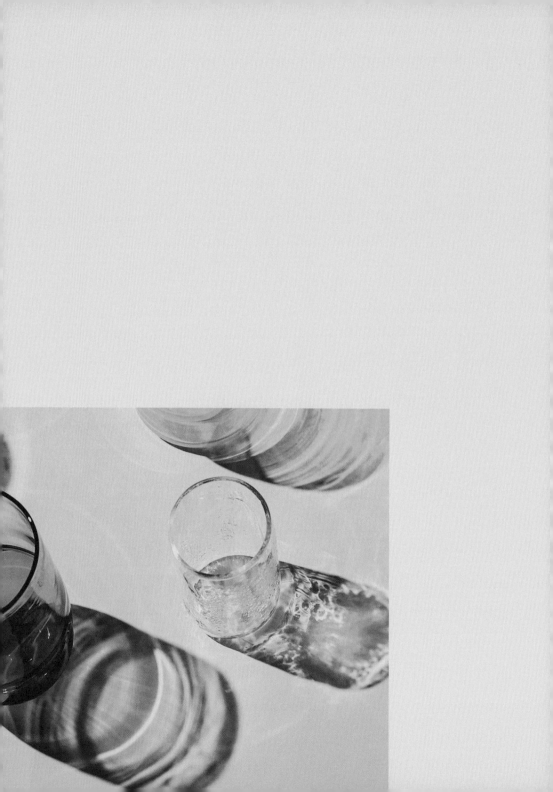

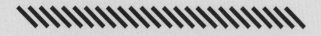

QUIZ

Why do you drink?

Maybe it's for lots of different reasons – or perhaps you're just not sure. It could be you just like feeling drunk? But once you know why you really drink, you'll understand far more clearly how to stop.

1 You've won a bottle of champagne. Do you open it:

a. Before a party, waiting for guests to arrive.
b. The night before a week you know will be tricky.
c. In bed, alone.
d. With friends, having also purchased a few more bottles.
e. On a weeknight when there's nothing on TV.
f. When you next have something to celebrate.

2 It's Friday, and you're at after-work drinks. Are you:

a. Knocking back a quick glass of wine at the bar before you join the others.
b. Ordering a full bottle for yourself – it's been a hellish week.
c. Starting on the shots. Why not?
d. Waiting to see what everyone else is drinking before you order.
e. Steadily drinking to cope with Karen from HR bleating on.
f. Having a medium-sized glass of wine and relaxing before you head home.

~~~~~~

3 You've just had a row with your partner and you need a drink. Do you:

a. Take a bottle of wine and lock yourself in the bathroom.

b. Pour a large whisky or gin and put a movie on.

c. Head for the pub. Sod it, several pubs.

d. WhatsApp your friends and beg them to meet you for drinks.

e. You don't need a drink, you're already buzzing (with rage).

f. Make a cup of tea – you don't feel like drinking.

4 You're at a wedding and you have to give a speech. Do you:

a. Down a large brandy beforehand.

b. Make sure everyone's glasses – including yours – are regularly topped up.

c. Down the contents of your hip flask in the loo.

d. Encourage everyone to share a drink with you before you begin.

e. Have a livener first, to make you wittier.

f. Wait until afterwards, then start on the wine.

5 Your friend wants a heart-to-heart. Do you meet:

a. In your kitchen, with wine.

b. In a noisy cocktail bar, with a plan to try them all.

c. In a variety of pubs and bars until somehow you're at a house party and it's 2am.

d. In a bar she likes, sharing the drinks she likes.

e. At hers, and you've brought two bottles.

f. In a café – maybe you'll go for a drink later.

6 You're going home for Christmas, where there will be tricky relatives. Do you:

a. Nip to the other room regularly for a secret slug of brandy.

b. Start on the Baileys on arrival.

c. Crack open the Christmas spirits, and keep going all night.

d. Bring several bottles and encourage everyone to join you.

e. Start drinking on the train – you need to prepare for this.

f. Agree to a Snowball, and save the big guns for New Year's Eve.

///

7 You're hosting a dinner party tonight. What's the drink situation?

a. You've started on the wine early, and are terrified of running out.

b. You're drinking while you cook, and laying out cocktail supplies for later.

c. You've bought ten bottles of wine, between four of you.

d. You've rung round to ask what people want to drink.

e. You've got aperitifs, wine, brandy and liqueurs.

f. You're putting the white in the fridge and looking forward to it.

8 You're drunk and having fun. Ideally, are you:

a. At a small party of close friends and family.

b. In a huge nightclub, dancing with tons of people.

c. Who cares? Could be anywhere.

d. At a glamorous dinner party.

e. On a yacht with a bunch of celebrities.

f. At a casual get-together in a friend's house.

Now add up your scores.
If you have a mix, then... well, you're a mix.

Mostly As: Anxious drinker

You tend to drink to cope with anxiety. For you, social occasions are stressful, and having a few drinks eases the tension. You're likely to knock a couple back before you set out, to steady your nerves, and when you're upset, a drink calms you down. The problem is it's hard to stop at one or two – as the buzz wears off, the nerves return and the paranoia of being publicly drunk kicks in. If you keep drinking, though, you've discovered you can ward off The Fear until the next day – when the hangover rolls in.

Mostly Bs: Distraction drinker

You drink mainly to take your mind off trouble. It instantly lifts your mood, diverts your attention and gives you a reason to enjoy yourself, rather than dwelling on whatever's going on in real life. Distraction is a habit, and you've found an instant way to relax and switch off your mind. But the difficulty is that you're just putting it off and the next day you'll still have to deal with the issue – but with a hangover this time.

Mostly Cs: Out-of-control drinker

Once you pop, you can't stop. You are drinking to chase the buzz, blot out unhappiness, relax, feel good and open up the possibility of a wild, wild night. Binge drinking means drowning your sorrows, worries and stresses in a lake of friendly booze. It also means you're storing up mental and physical health problems, and you're much more likely to be making bad decisions – either when drunk, or in the throes of regret afterwards.

Mostly Ds: Crowd-pleasing drinker

You are a go-with-the-flow type. Your friends like drinking, so it's easy to knock it back along with them. When you're home alone, you're not too bothered – but when you're out and everyone else is having double JD and Coke, then so are you. And if your best friend suggests another round at midnight, you're not going to be the one to spoil the party. Equally, if your partner opens a bottle, it'd be rude not to share it over dinner. Your drinking is sociable – but if your life is too, you can easily end up drunk every night.

Mostly Es: Bored drinker

You don't get a huge amount of joy from everyday life – and drinking eases the boredom. Maybe you don't have many friends who get your jokes, or you're in a relationship that's going nowhere. Perhaps your job is uninspiring, but you don't know how to change things. Drinking puts you in a different headspace, makes you feel part of things and gives you a purpose. When you're drunk, you don't have to confront the aspects of your life that you dislike – but the trouble is, they don't go away.

Mostly Fs: Enjoyment drinker

You just like drinking. It tastes good, being a bit drunk feels nice, it's a sociable thing to do and besides, who wants to be the person sipping tonic water when everyone else is having a riotous time? You don't think you have a problem, and you would never describe yourself as a binge drinker – but you do sometimes think you should cut down a bit. The truth is, though, 'binge drinking' means just six units in one session – and you can sink more than that over a quiet chat in your friend's kitchen. It might be useful to look at why you enjoy drinking so much – and whether it's simply become a habit.

What if it's serious?

If none of the aforementioned quite fits, but you struggle to manage life without alcohol, you may be in danger of alcoholism. Think about whether you are:

/ **Drinking a lot, but don't get drunk easily.**

/ **Drunk after a couple of glasses, but just carrying on.**

/ **Needing a drink to get going in the morning.**

/ **Finding the idea of an evening or weekend without a drink horrific.**

/ **Struggling to manage your life and relationships.**

/ **Getting ill and feeling hungover and always below par.**

/ **Making self-destructive choices.**

/ **Drinking to hide depression, guilt, grief or other negative, painful emotions.**

If so, you are using alcohol to self-medicate. There are issues in your life or your past that are just too hard to deal with without booze, but they won't resolve while you're drinking. So either:

/ **Go to your doctor and ask for help with quitting alcohol.**

/ **Go to an AA meeting; they are held all over the place every night, so there will always be one within reach all over the world. Visit alcoholics-anonymous.org.uk to find out more.**

/ **Find a registered therapist who specialises in addiction issues.**

It's tempting just to ask friends and family to support you, but that's asking a lot if you don't also have professional help. Many people find it too hard to watch somebody struggle with addiction without judging, criticising or taking on their problems. That's why professional help is so valuable. Doctors, AA sponsors and therapists are not there to judge you – they are the first step towards helping you get better.

Now you know what type of drinker you are, you can start to unravel the reasons behind your drinking, and tackle your habits in a way that will work for you.

Anxious drinker

You need to feel more confident. Whether you're shy, socially anxious, suffer from panic attacks or all of those things, you will need to find a way to replicate the feeling of certainty and sudden assurance that alcohol gives you. The upside of this is that alcohol wears off, whereas real confidence doesn't.

Things to try:

Keep a diary of your triggers / look for patterns, such as bad sleep, a hangover or stress at work. Knowing where it begins can help you find coping techniques for those situations.

Learn breathing techniques / being able to trip your body into relaxing is an invaluable tool. Find videos of what to do on YouTube.

See your doctor about counselling / if your anxiety is specific (crowds, planes), CBT (cognitive behavioural therapy) or EMDR (eye movement desensitisation and reprocessing) can be very helpful, with fast results. If you suffer from GAD (generalised anxiety disorder), you may also benefit from therapy and anti-anxiety tablets such as beta blockers or Citalopram.

Exercise / I don't want to sound like your old PE teacher, but a session in the gym, yoga, swimming, a run or a brisk walk in nature all really help to regulate anxiety and calm you down. Many people find that regular exercise is all they need to cope.

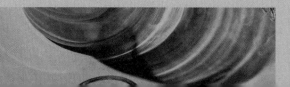

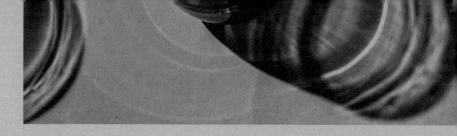

Distraction drinker

You need to figure out what you're avoiding. Whether it's work or money issues, relationship difficulties or just general dissatisfaction with life, once you begin to confront the problems, you can start to solve them. Even if they seem to you insurmountable.

Things to try:

Get advice / for practical issues – debt, relationships, work problems – there are organisations that can help you. Stepchange for debt advice (stepchange.org), the Citizen's Advice Bureau (citizensadvice.org.uk) and Relate (relate.org. uk) all have global equivalents wherever you are, and will give you non-judgmental advice.

Talk to friends / a problem shared really can be a problem halved – you may worry that they'll judge you, but you might well be pleasantly surprised by how helpful it is just to have somebody listen to you.

Make a list / grit your teeth and work out what the foundations of the problem are – how much debt you're in, what the real trouble is in your relationship or why you aren't happy at work. Once you know what's going on, it's easier to tackle it step by step and start making good decisions.

Out-of-control drinker

You're in danger of addiction – or you may be already there. Though you know your drinking is dangerous, and regularly puts you in risky situations, you can't stop. You need to examine what's driving your helter-skelter approach to booze.

Things to try:

Therapy / via your doctor or privately. A few sessions with a good psychotherapist can uncover the reasons behind your approach to drinking.

A total break / you need a major reset, so consider a few days away somewhere, drinkfree, with supportive friends, if that's possible.

Go to an AA meeting / it's not just for long-term alcoholics. AA offers a non-judgmental, supportive 'safe space' to talk about your drinking (see page 29).

Join an alcohol-free activity / if all your friends are enabling you, and drinking just as much, consider doing voluntary work or joining a class or an organisation such as Club Soda (joinclubsoda.co.uk), which holds regular events for non-drinkers.

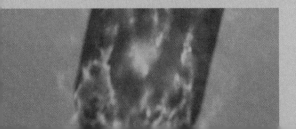

Crowd-pleasing drinker

You hate the idea of standing out – your friends drink, and the idea of being the buzzkill makes you cringe. Having to say 'not for me' and explain why, having people think you might be an alcoholic in recovery… it's easier just to keep drinking, even when you know you've had enough.

Things to try:

Change the circumstances / daytime activities, a cinema trip, a gig instead of a bar can all break the habit.

Lie / if you really struggle to say no, just say you're on antibiotics, and if anyone asks what for, tell them it's for a gum infection. While not normally advocating fibs, it can be easier when you're in a large group of keen drinkers.

Ask yourself if you're really enjoying every drink / if you're drinking for the sake of it, a little mindfulness goes a long way. Swap every second drink for a sparkling water with lime instead.

Don't do rounds / just say you're saving money, so you can be in charge of your own drinks, rather than having your evening set by whoever's knocking it back the fastest.

Bored drinker

When you're drinking because the alternative is boredom, there's no incentive to stop, other than your health and the chance to get to the bottom of what's really causing the problem. The aim is to break the boredom cycle.

Things to try:

Don't go out / for a week, or even a fortnight – long enough to notice what's really going on in your life without the reward of a pint or a bottle with pals.

Keep a diary / noting when you're particularly craving alcohol, and what else is going on to make you feel uncomfortable sober. Be aware of how hard alcohol is being sold to you as a solution to discomfort and boredom – TV shows, movies, adverts – and notice your responses to images of booze.

Replace your alcohol rituals / with an alternative 'reward', such as a relaxing early evening bath, a glass of Seedlip (non-alcoholic distilled spirit) or a mocktail (see pages 114–131).

Enjoyment drinker

It may be that you drink for mentally healthy reasons: you just like to relax after a tough day; you only have a good bottle of red on a Friday; you're just having fun with friends. But as you get older, all the fun reasons for drinking become less important than whether your drinking is harming you. And if you're drinking more than you intend, or way over the recommended limit, it's time to address the issue.

Things to try:

Stock up on alternatives / it's very easy to crack open wine when it's all you've got in the fridge. Invest in alcohol-free wine and beer, now available at most supermarkets.

Figure out how much you're spending on alcohol / do a rough monthly tally and think about saving the same amount for a week away or something else you really want.

Hold a lunchtime get-together / with Virgin Marys and mocktails (see pages 114–131) instead of a dinner party, or go to a pub quiz where the focus is on the questions, not the drinking, and stay on soft drinks.

Be the designated driver / people will be grateful, and it's a perfect excuse not to join in.

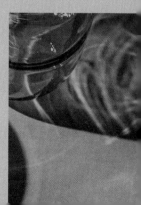

What's stoppin me?

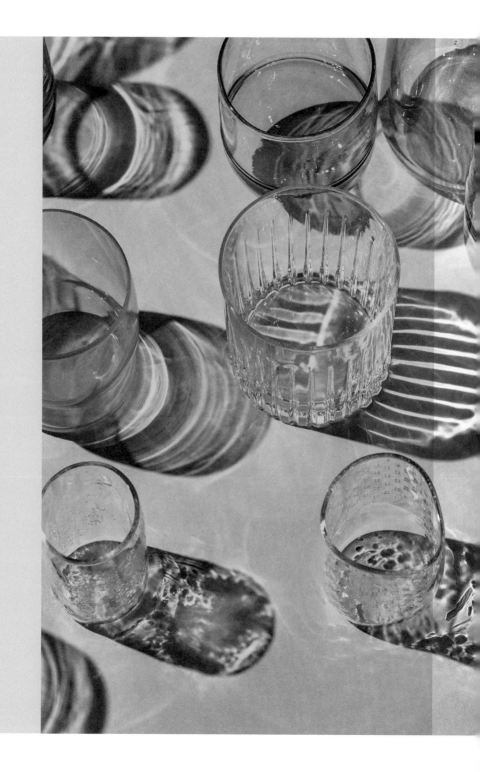

The fear around quitting

Fear is at the core of everything difficult in life. Think about giving up, and there'll be a fear buried somewhere (or maybe it's already shining out, like the Statue of Liberty after a good polish). Giving up alcohol – and even significantly cutting down – can trigger all of the buried stuff you don't like to think about. It may feel as though quitting will just open the floodgates to all the unpleasant thoughts you shoved in a box marked 'do not open' and kicked under the bed.

Then there are the more obvious fears, directly related to giving up. Here are some common ones...

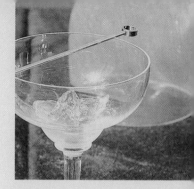

Will I lose my friends?

If your main social engagement with your friends involves drinking, it's not surprising that you don't want to be the odd one out. What will you talk about when you're sober? Will they still invite you out – and will you actually still find them interesting?

The truth is, you might lose a few pals. Friendships that are based solely on the mutual interest of drinking may fall by the wayside. But the real friendships will actually improve. You'll quickly find that being sober makes it easy to tell who you really like – and who you're just hanging out with for the sake of it, or because you always have done. Removing the fog of alcohol means you can see the people around you clearly for the first time in years. Worried about what you'll talk about? The same things you've always talked about – and more interesting things too. And if they don't invite you out, that's because they think you'll judge them for drinking, or because 'there's no point' if you're not boozing. Think about that: if a night out is pointless when it's not oiled by ethanol, what was the point in the first place?

As for whether they'll be interesting – if they're interesting people, of course they will be.

What if I don't have fun any more?

The idea that 'boozefree = boring' is deeply entrenched in society. Any depiction of friends together having a laugh means beer for men, wine for women, cocktails for young people, whisky for old people... the dread of dullness is what keeps many of us knocking it back.

But if the only route to fun is being drunk, you may be hanging out with the wrong people. Or maybe sometimes you're drinking because it whisks away your inhibitions like a magician with a tablecloth, allowing you to make jokes, be the life and soul, flirt, have wild sex – all the things you feel unable to do when sober. If that's the case, it's useful to look at why you feel you can't allow yourself to let go, without the drink giving you permission. Whether it's shyness, social anxiety or self-loathing, where you need drink to actually like yourself, a course of therapy could be very useful in helping you approach life without that crippling self-consciousness.

How will I celebrate?

Weddings, birthdays, Christmas, New Year, babies, new jobs… everything except passing your driving test (and even then) is associated with drinking. So how are you going to mark the occasion without a shot / flute / glass / bottle?

'Drink = celebration' is an assumption, not a fact. But it's been exploited by advertising like a 1930s child star. There is no rule stating that marriage means champagne, or finishing your finals means doing shots, or that Christmas is no fun without Baileys. Yet it's entrenched in our minds that in order to mark a rite of passage, alcohol must be heavily involved, from 'wetting the baby's head' (like the baby knows or cares) to toasting the deceased at a funeral (like they know or care). Marking an occasion is about who you're with, not what you're drinking – and if you must have sneezy bubbles up your nose, no-alcohol prosecco is nowadays virtually indistinguishable from the real thing.

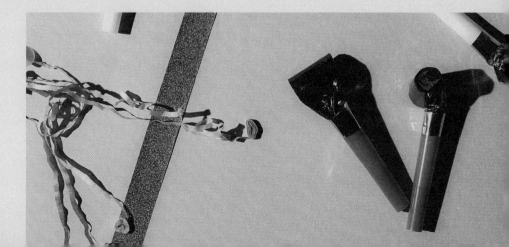

How will I relax?

It's an instant destresser and a friend in need… as every birthday card aimed at mothers claims, we're all counting down to 'wine o'clock', while any stressed-sounding social media post is met with, 'Pour yourself a big glass of wine, hun.' Is it even possible to calm down without it after a tough day? Anything tricky, challenging or scary is made immediately easier with a stiff drink – or so we've been led to believe. When you're required to step up – for a speech, presentation or exam – drink is a speedy anxiety-quencher.

Yes, drink does relax you at first. But over time it messes with your brain's neurotransmitters, making it more likely that you'll feel anxious or depressed. So while you're relaxed in the short term, you're adding to a Jenga pile of anxiety in the long term, plus delicately placing the hangover-regret and stupid-drunk-decision likelihood on top of that wobbly pile. Instead, there are many relaxation techniques you can learn to use before a test of courage…

Hypnotherapy / a session with a qualified therapist can fix exam anxiety.

Breathing / hold one nostril shut and count your breath: four in through the other nostril, then four out through the mouth. Reverse nostrils and carry on until you feel calmer.

Massage your earlobe / it's an acupressure point that can help to calm your breathing and lower your heart rate.

Lie down / and tense and release every muscle in your body, from your feet upwards.

Sing / loudly.

Exercise / a session at the gym or a brisk walk releases endorphins and calms you down. Or dance to some loud and lovely music.

Creativity / once your focus is on taking the photograph, arranging the scrapbook or starting the novel, you won't be as fixated on the upcoming dread.

Get a pet / therapy pets are scientifically proven to help with anxiety. Stroking a cat or dog can lower blood pressure and reduce your heart rate, and walking a dog is excellent for managing stress.

Feel the fear and do it anyway / seriously, nobody ever died of fear. Except in horror stories.

How will I meet anyone?

Dating can be terrifying. Having to struggle through the small talk, worry about what they think of you, then – oh God – sex with a new person… would anyone ever form a relationship at all, if it weren't for alcohol?

Of course it's scary, meeting a whole new person – particularly after a tough break-up or a divorce. The idea of polite conversation, working out if they're mad, letting someone see your nakedness with fresh eyes… of course you need a drink. Except you don't. Assessing whether you want to date someone again is far better done sober, because after five glasses of wine and a shot, he or she looks like the best bet in the world. Of course you should go back to theirs! Of course you should have crazy, new sex and creep out at 4am to call a cab! Of course you should wake up the next day and wonder what their name was and how that happened and why you didn't use protection…

Sober dating is initially unnerving, for sure. But really, so is drunk dating. Just grit your teeth and do it. If they're right for you, the conversation will flow when you're sober too.

How will I cope with tough times?

Break-ups, bereavement, job loss, illness… maybe you think you'll manage okay without drink when times are good – but you can't imagine life without an alcohol crutch when they're bad. Everyone gets drunk when they're sad, right?

It is such a common response to trauma; every other TV drama features a lonely woman knocking back white wine, or a newly divorced man cracking open the whisky. But drinking when you're down will never, ever cheer you up. Yes, there might be a false rush of hope, a sparkling burst of prosecco-fuelled sentiment and optimism. But an hour later, you're on the long, dark slope to despair, because alcohol is a depressant. You'll keep drinking to chase the high (but it's long gone, I promise you) or you'll keep drinking to oblivion. And that's a) terribly bad for your mind and body, and b) going to result in a hangover like a medieval painting of hell. Drink is not your friend in the bad times. Your friends are your friends – so turn to them, not the bottle.

What will it do to my relationship?

If you and your partner rely on alcohol to communicate, and it's an ongoing third party in your coupledom, one of you quitting can tear the wheels right off. No more cosy nights with a bottle or three, no more uninhibited sex… you may as well split up.

Admittedly, it's far tougher to quit or dramatically cut down when your partner is merrily pouring a fourth glass of merlot and you're sipping sparkling water. I know, because that was my situation. Not only is it a temptation, it also means that after a few, your partner will be on a different planet. Planet not-making-much-sense. Planet you're-so-boring-nowadays. Planet come-on-let's-go-over-to-Dave's when you're knackered and want to go to bed. So if you can quit together, it's easier.

If not, however, it can still be done. Just make an agreement that if you're out and your other half is drunk while you are sober, you're allowed to go home when you need to. The last thing you need is drunken pressure to stay and 'have fun'. At home, equally agree that when you need to go to bed, you will – if your pissed partner wants to stay up playing obscure nineties rap, or watching cat videos on YouTube, they can. But you don't have to join in.

And if you not drinking brings up a lot of difficult issues – that's not about the drink. It's about the relationship.

I can't sleep without it

Sleep can be elusive – and many of us rely on a nip or three
of something to get to sleep in the first place. Without your
evening wine or your bedtime nightcap, how will you manage
your life?

Here's the truth, though: booze can help you get to sleep
initially, but it disrupts your sleeping patterns. You spend
less time in restorative REM sleep and are much more
likely to wake up sweating at 4am, feeling like a crumbling
parchment scroll through dehydration. Alcohol is also a
diuretic, so you'll be up and down to the loo, dehydrating
yourself further. None of this adds up to a good night's
sleep, which is partly why you feel so exhausted with a
hangover. It's because you are. Instead, try the following
for a better night's sleep…

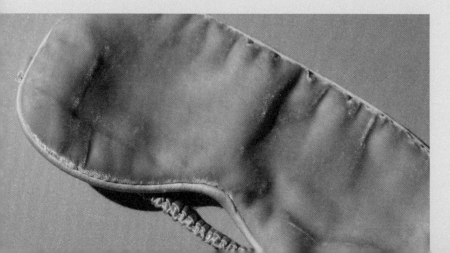

Don't fight it / if you can't sleep, accept it. There's no point lying there raging and fretting. Get up, make a cup of herbal tea, read a book. It will come eventually.

Sort your bedroom out / declutter your space, get some fresh air into the room and keep a glass of water by the bed. Tidy bedroom, tidy mind.

Sort snoring out / if your partner snores, kick them off to the doctor and invest in silicone earplugs (they are life-changing).

If worries are keeping you awake / write down everything that's bothering you, and leave it in another room to look at tomorrow. Sounds odd, but it works.

Have a warm bath before bed / a shower will wake you up, whereas a bath will soothe you to sleep.

Read, but don't watch TV or go on social media / blue screen light triggers wakefulness, so turn your phone off and open a book instead.

Take medication / if insomnia is an ongoing problem, herbal or non-herbal sleeping pills might be an answer for a while. Have a chat with your doctor – and stop self-medicating with the drinks cupboard.

Fight the fear

There may be other reasons why you're scared to give up too – for lots of us, it's just the vague feeling that life without the sparkle and uplift of alcohol will be a monotonous drift, with fewer lows, but no highs either.

It's very easy to let your dread of the negative consequences of quitting stop you trying to quit at all. But if you accept that there might be a few downsides at first, but that the positives will outweigh them, you can overcome any reason you can think of to keep on boozing. Here's how to tackle the fear straight away…

Write a list / of the positives of quitting FOR YOU, not just generic ones that could apply to everyone and no one. Then print it out and stick it on the fridge, or somewhere you'll see it regularly.

Plan ahead / don't suddenly decide to do this two weeks before Christmas, or throw out all the half-empty bottles on a whim. Choose a date for stopping and put it in your diary. On that day, make sure the house is free of all booze.

Tell people you trust / but don't tell everyone yet. If you know you'll get support, confide – but any friends who are going to hassle you to 'just have one' really don't need to be involved at this stage.

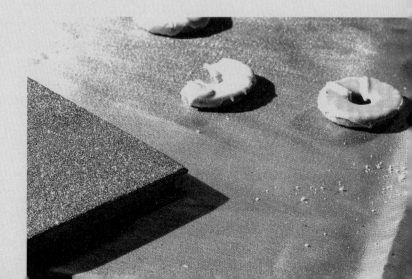

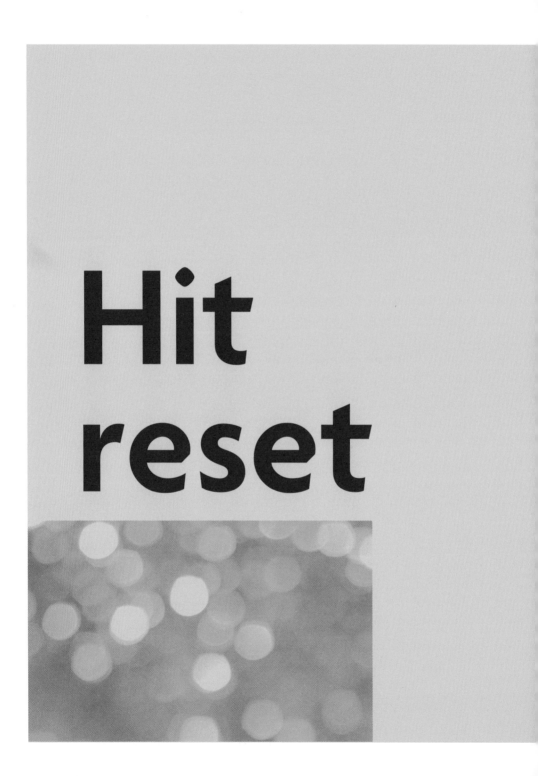

Hit reset

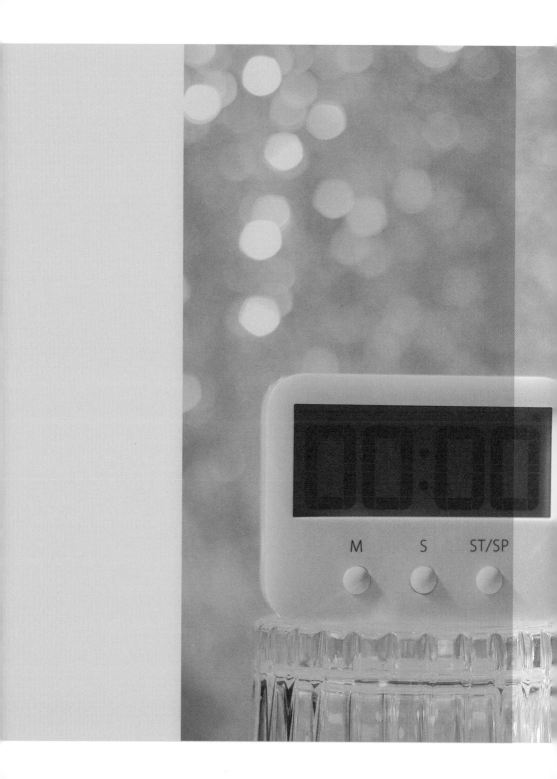

///

You know you want to stop, or significantly cut down.
You've faced down your own fear, and you understand the
following truths:

/ Drinking is affecting your life in a negative way.

**/ Drink is just ethanol – a poisonous chemical – mixed
with flavouring and a great deal of advertising money.**

**/ A severe hangover is not a small price to pay for a great
night out; it's your body desperately trying to process
and eject poison.**

/ If you like people, you'll like them both drunk or sober.

/ If you don't, you'll just realise faster that they're idiots.

**/ You will like yourself more when you aren't making
drunken / hungover decisions.**

/ You'll save money.

/ You can drive to places and leave whenever you want.

But while knowing all this stuff is very helpful, actually doing it is a different matter. You are going against years of conditioning – years of being told that:

/ **You can't have fun without a drink.**

/ **Drinking makes you feel good, instantly.**

/ **Going out = drinking.**

/ **Drink will cheer you up.**

/ **Drink will calm you down.**

/ **You must drink to celebrate.**

/ **You must drink to commiserate.**

/ **Drinking wine with dinner is sophisticated.**

/ **Drinking cocktails is exciting and glamorous.**

/ **Drinking beer is friendly and enjoyable.**

/ **Drinking gin is what mums do after a tough day.**

/ **Drinking beer is what men do to bond with friends.**

And on and on and on. Go into any greetings card shop and you'll find card after card making nudge-wink jokes about drinking. Unlike overeating or taking drugs, drinking a lot carries no social stigma whatsoever, even though it's just as bad – or worse – for you: more likely to end in violence, and more likely to turn into a lifelong problem. Yes, the Western world is in denial. But you don't have to be.

Getting started

Some think that if you want to quit, you have to quit forever. Last drink, no more, teetotal till the end of time. But while this may be the only option for alcoholics, for those who just want a break or to give their livers a rest for a while, it's a bit extreme. Plus, telling yourself you can never drink again is guaranteed to make you fantasize wildly about alcohol and all the joy and happiness you'll never feel again. So pick a timescale – a month, six months, a year – and tell yourself you'll reassess when that time is up. Most people, having realised how much easier life is without booze, don't return to it. But you might want to have a glass of champagne at weddings, or a whisky at New Year, or the occasional glass of wine. The main thing is that you're resetting your attitude to alcohol and how you consume it; to do that, you really need at least three months.

Yes, Dry January and Sober October can be very useful for your liver (and raise money for charity), but four weeks is just enough time to start getting used to it, then before you know it, it's over. So if you can, think in seasons, not months.

First things first: set a date and stick to it. Like quitting smoking, it's useful to get rid of any leftover alcohol in the house, so you won't feel tempted. Of course, you can always go out and buy more – but by the time you've put your jacket on, you may have talked yourself out of it.

If you just want to cut down, rather than quit, it's still a very good plan to cut it out altogether for a few weeks. It gives you a chance to view life without the hazy lens of nightly wine, and look at what's bothering you, what you might be using alcohol for and how much you really want to give up. If you don't have a period without it, it's easy to cut down for a few days, then slip gradually back into your normal drinking patterns.

Some people find a goal helps – getting married (though I'm not suggesting you do this just to stay sober), running a marathon, losing weight, saving money – if it's something you can work towards, and you know not drinking is part of achieving that, it's more likely to keep you on track.

Tips

to help you on your way

For the first few days or weeks, if you're used to drinking every night (or most nights, or days), you need to make it as easy as possible on yourself. Here's how…

Chuck out the booze

If you're giving up smoking, you don't carry a battered pack around in your pocket, just in case. (Or if you do, that's why it hasn't worked.) So having white wine in the fridge 'for guests' or a cocktail cabinet of weird holiday liqueurs is an absolute guarantee that at some point you'll decide a small one won't hurt. Throw them out. Don't think of it as a waste of money – think of it as chucking a whole bunch of nauseous hangovers down the sink.

If your partner or housemate still drinks...

If they aren't quitting along with you, there will be booze. You could ask them to drink something you really don't like for a week or so (for instance, there is nothing about cans of warm bitter or a flinty sauvignon that appeals to me). But if you like everything, designate a section of the fridge or cupboard 'X's booze shelf' and tell yourself that having any would be stealing. It is not your booze.

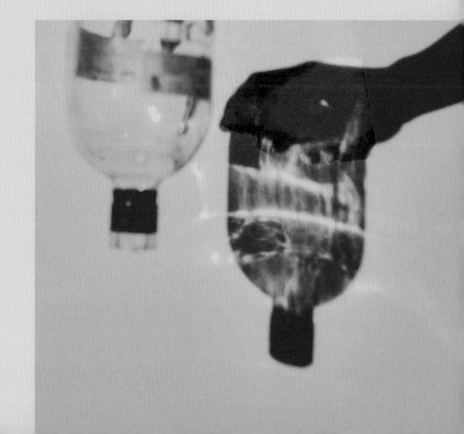

Don't go out

No, really. Bars, restaurants, friends' houses – they're all drinking triggers. The exception is the theatre or cinema – but that's expensive. I suggest downloading a few immersive box sets, like *The Sopranos*, *Breaking Bad*, *Spiral*, *The Bridge* – anything that will take your mind off sociable drinking and fill up an evening.

Reward yourself

After a long day, it's natural to want a drink. So stock up on other rewards instead – non-alcoholic drinks like Seedlip (see mocktails on pages 114–131), expensive hot chocolate or fancy tea or coffee. Or promise yourself a country walk, a new book, an hour in a hot bath, an uninterrupted podcast… It has to be something you'll look forward to so that the evening doesn't slip away leaving you bored and unfulfilled.

Find a 'sober buddy'

Maybe a friend is quitting too – or you know someone who stopped a while ago. Having a person you can call or text for support when you're craving a drink can make all the difference. In AA these are known as 'sponsors' (see page 27), but even if you're just trying to manage your wine habit a bit, having someone to call who isn't murmuring 'you're no fun any more' can be a huge help.

Change your routine

If you always go for a drink on Fridays, or you and your partner like to open a bottle of wine on a Saturday night, don't try and do the same thing, but just without booze – do something altogether different for a while. Go bowling or to the cinema, visit a booze-free café for an early dinner, watch TV while you eat, try making mocktails (see pages 114–131), go for a long walk with sandwiches and a Thermos of tea… yes, your weekend may be a bit like a sheltered 15-year-old's weekend in 1956, but that's no bad thing. They had fun too, you know.

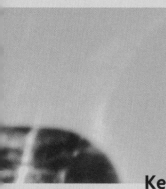

Keep a diary

Not a 'Dear Diary, today I didn't drink again' kind of diary, but one that is purely for noting triggers. So if you're struggling, write down when the craving strikes. Was it when you discovered your ex was dating again? When you came in starving and couldn't be bothered to cook? When your housemate poured a big glass of pinot? All of the above? Knowing what drives your desire to drink is key to being able to distract yourself at the right moment, and plan ahead for when the triggers strike.

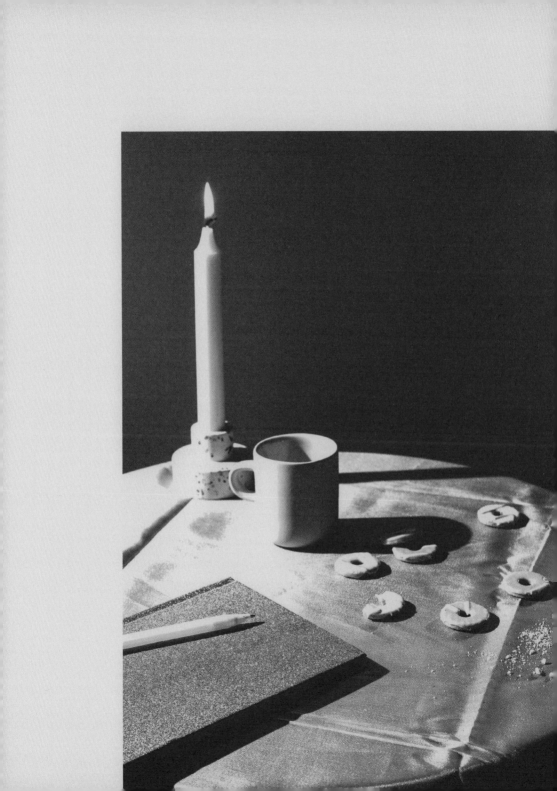

What to say to your friends

It's vital to have a story – an explanation – that will shut down persuasion, moaning, excessive questioning and argument about your decision not to drink, at least until your friends have accepted it as your normal and shut up about it. See below for some easy fibs to have at the ready, as well as some other ways you can get round any interrogation.

'I'm on antibiotics.'
Downside: This won't work for very long.

'I'm driving.'
Downside: You will actually have to drive, always, and will end up giving everyone a lift home, ten miles in the wrong direction.

'I'm feeling a bit ill.'
Downside: You'll be met with 'A drink will cheer you up' and you can't be ill forever.

'I'm saving money.'
Downside: Someone will offer to buy you a drink.

'I've already got myself a G&T.'
Downside: A glass of sparkling water with a slice of lime can look exactly like a G&T and deter questions – until someone buys you another, or asks for a sip.

Have a look at what you could say instead – and be prepared for some of these responses:

You

'I'm not drinking at the moment, to give my body a break. I wasn't really enjoying it enough to make the hangovers worth it.'

Them

'You're obviously drinking the wrong things – try this wine.'
'It's always worth it!'
'But you'll be back on it for the wedding / Christmas / my 30th, right?'

You

'I really need a break from it at the moment. I don't know if it's a permanent decision, but I'm feeling much better without it for now.' (Aim for firm, friendly and brief.)

Them

'But don't you miss drinking?'

You

'Not yet, but I'm sure there will be times when I'll miss it a bit.'

They will almost certainly add, 'Well, I couldn't do it.'

There is no answer to this that isn't either smug, judge-y or a lie. Just smile and change the subject.

Don't...

Be judgmental / 'You should try cutting down too; you do drink quite a lot', won't work for anyone.

Bang on / 'I just found that it was affecting my mental health, and what with the break-up and the new job, I thought I really couldn't carry on the way I was.' (Note: This is fine if someone asks – but if they don't, keep it brief.)

Downplay it / 'Oh, I'll probably be back on it by next week, I've got no willpower, your wine looks great…' This just undermines your decisions and gives people permission to persuade you.

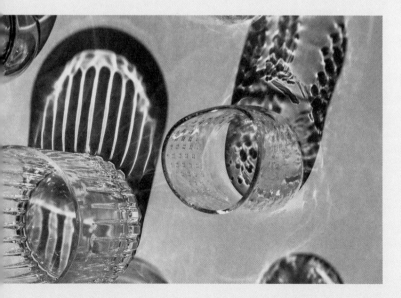

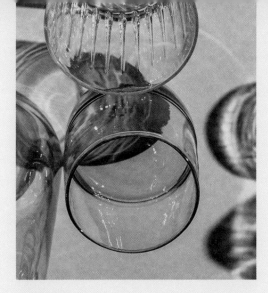

Criticise other people's routes to sobriety / 'AA is so over the top, I'm doing it with no help at all, it's ridiculous to call drinking an illness…' You have no idea what has led other people to their own sobriety – so respect their choices, even if they're not your own.

Be evangelical / 'I just feel so different – so wide awake, it's like a new world, everyone should try it, I'm getting so much done, I've started running…' Nobody likes a preacher. Keep it to yourself until specifically asked.

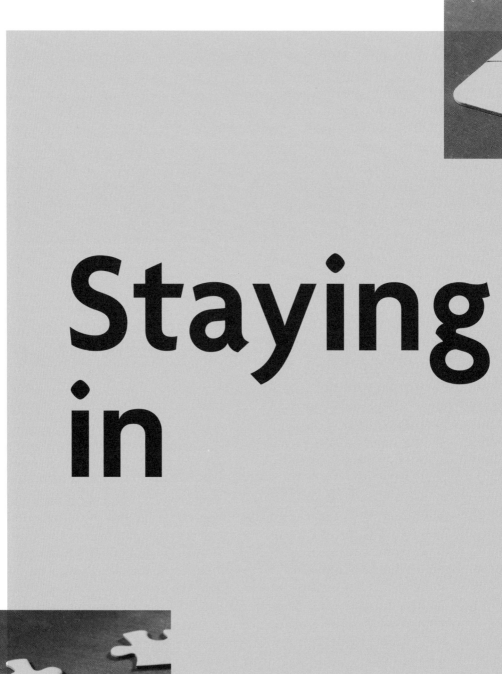

Staying in

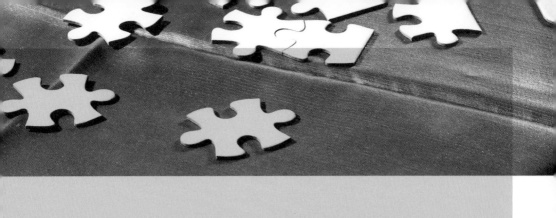

Pretty much every dating profile ever goes along the lines of: 'As happy going out for cocktails as I am staying in, curled up on the sofa with a bottle of red!' But what if you don't do either – and your sofa time is now all about the peppermint tea and the Evian?

Staying in is almost always portrayed by the media as 'cosy' – and that means (apparently) drinking, alone or with your partner. I can't think of a film where a character went to someone's house in the evening without a glass of wine being poured, or a group of male friends got together without beer. It's a constant bombardment: Netflix means wine, football means beer, a date coming round means prosecco or champagne, a long day with the kids or sitting in the garden in summer means a G&T, a dinner party means bring wine, an open fire equals whisky. We've absorbed these messages all our lives and it's no wonder that for many of us, 'staying in and relaxing' means 'opening a bottle of something'.

‰‰

And the fact is, sometimes staying in is boring. You're home from work, there's nothing on TV apart from smug house-y programmes and more grim news – how else are you going to relax? Whether you live alone and enjoy a quiet glass of wine, or with a partner and share a take-the-day-off drink when you get in, or with housemates who are always up for cracking open a beer while you cook, alcohol goes hand in hand with 'staying in and relaxing'.

Of course, it may not be every night – sometimes maybe you're at the gym, or you're feeling too tired, or you're working late – but if you are someone who, like I was, associates 'relax' with 'drink', it can be tricky to do 'cosy night in' without 'cosy glass of instant soother'.

But it is possible – and here's how...

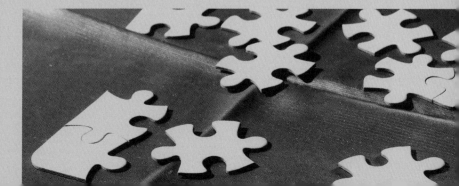

Move
the booze

If you live with a partner, or in a shared house, you cutting down or quitting doesn't mean everyone is doing the same – so there's still going to be booze around. Rituals are borne from habits, and if your habit is to open the fridge, grasp the white wine from the door and pour yourself a large one, it's very hard to ignore it whenever you open the fridge around 6pm. Likewise, the gin on your charming retro drinks trolley, or the beer you keep on the middle shelf. Whatever you're used to doing is probably what you're going to keep on doing – unless you make a noticeable change. So…

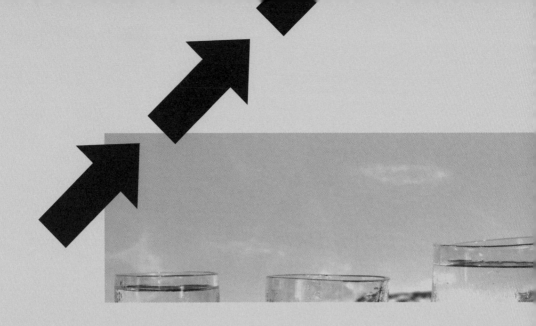

Ask if the drinkers can:

Move the wine to a different part of the fridge /
and keep it in a bag. It may sound a bit excessive, but if you don't see the cold condensing on the green glass, and recall that chilled, flinty first sip as a result, your reptilian brain won't instantly be triggered to ditch all previous plans and knock it back.

Keep the beer in a non-food cupboard /
so that it's not laughing in your face every time you go to get a packet of pasta out.

Agree to retire the drinks trolley /
cabinet or shelf until you're used to not drinking. And in the place where the booze used to be, put a very nice soft drink (or a selection), so that when your hand automatically reaches out, it lands on something alcohol free.

Change the habit

Nowhere triggers habits more than your own home, and if your usual pattern is to come in from work, heave a sigh, chuck your jacket on a chair and pour yourself a drink (or get the kids in bed, heave a sigh, etc.), you will decide you're not drinking, come in from work, do the sighing and jacket-chucking and then your brain will light up like a fruit machine, with a row of wine glasses clunking into place. Basically, we are all Pavlov's dogs, entirely conditioned to do what we always do, and then do it some more, because having-wine-when-we-expect-wine makes the reward areas of our primitive brains light up and jingle and play an electronic tune. If we do all the same things but then tell ourselves we can't have it, the happy tune fast becomes a plaintive wail of loss, echoing through a burned-out building. Which is why you need to change the habit before it begins.

Here are some things you can do at your normal 'drinking time' instead:

/ Go for a shower or bath, and change your clothes for the evening.

/ Go for a walk.

/ Pick up your current book and read a chapter.

/ Spend a few minutes catching up or posting on social media.

/ Take some pictures in the garden or outside.

/ Put some music on and have a little dance.

/ Call someone on the phone.

/ Meditate, with or without an app like Headspace.

/ Write down your thoughts and feelings in a journal.

/ Make yourself a fancy mocktail (see pages 114–131).

/ Have a scroll through Netflix, or whatever streaming service you have, and pick something to watch later on that you can look forward to. Old DVDs are good too (and very cheap in local charity shops).

/ Do a quick, easy workout.

/ Have a jigsaw on the go (make it a 1,000-piece one, at least).

/ Play on Xbox.

/ Start knitting or crafting, to keep your hands busy.

Whatever you do for distraction, have a large drink of water. No, it doesn't have the social cachet of a large glass of merlot, but all too often you're 'dying for a drink' because you're just thirsty, and you associate alcohol with feeling better. Water will sort out the thirsty part and liven you up a bit, before you get on with your evening.

Tune in to your emotions

Alongside habit, a major reason for drinking at home is to tweak emotions. So whether you're feeling fed up, irritated, depressed, down, weary, nervous or any other word in the thesaurus of negative feelings, you've come to believe that a drink will fix it and return you to 'fairly happy, all things considered'.

And it might – for a bit – but you still feel the same underneath. You've just poured some Happy Juice on top, and fairly soon it's going to wear off. In therapy, they're big on 'feeling your feelings' and not coshing them with chemicals. If you don't feel them, they will leak out in other ways – resentment, depression, anger… all the fun stuff.

The key to dealing with emotions as they arise is to work out what they are; otherwise when you feel something negative and just chuck booze at it, you turn it into a vague soup of misery without ever really knowing what it's about, and therefore being able to deal with it and find a solution.

A good place to start is HALT. They use this handy acronym in AA, and it stands for Hungry, Angry, Lonely, Tired. Of course, you could be feeling all four at the same time. But when you suddenly find yourself craving a drink, halt everything and ask yourself the following questions…

Am I hungry?

Hunger is guaranteed to make you feel bad-tempered, panicky and dissatisfied. If you have low blood sugar due to not having eaten for a while, it's tempting to chuck back an alcoholic drink to reset your faint, fading brain and relax you. Step away until you have done a quick feeling audit and figured out if you are craving carbs rather than booze. Quick fixes include nuts, wholegrain toast, fruit or crackers… and OK, yes, chocolate if it's an emergency.

Am I angry?

Anger is a difficult and painful feeling; if you're feeling it, it's no wonder you want to make it stop, and hope the quickest way is to throw some alcohol at it and make it go away. But although a drink may defer it, it won't erase it.

Instead, tell a friend. Or write it down. Or go and smash plates in the garden (then sweep them up, as you don't want hedgehogs tripping over your broken crockery). Try deep breathing or meditating too. Or – controversial – tell the person you're angry with why you're angry. Better out than in, usually.

Am I lonely?

If you live alone, or everyone is out, or away, or you've just gone through a break-up, or your best friend has moved to Canberra, you may be dying for a drink just so that you feel less alone. Alcohol can temporarily create a buffer zone around sadness and lift your flagging spirits. But loneliness is a condition you can change, rather than a feeling to euthanise. Make a call, send a message, ask yourself who (and what) you need in your life, and you can begin to change the feeling. Alcohol will just add self-pity on top of loneliness.

Am I tired?

We're all tired. And when you've had a long day of work, or kids, or caring, or just everything all at once, it's likely that the obvious way to wake yourself up is with a drink. (That's why they used to call it 'a livener'.) As it hits your bloodstream, you get a rush of sudden energy, a lift of the spirits and a feeling of relief. The trouble is that it's a fake feeling – it wears off as soon as you start enjoying it, and then the only answer is to drink some more to chase the good feeling, forgetting that alcohol is a depressant and will make you more tired as the evening wears on. It'll also screw with your sleep later, ensuring you wake up double tired the next day.

If you're tired, you can:

/ **Drink more water (dehydration can cause extreme tiredness).**
/ **Eat something low GI to give you some steady energy (pulses, fruit and whole grains).**
/ **Go for a walk – you may be in need of fresh air.**
/ **Have a shower.**
/ **Have a coffee.**
/ **Have a disco nap for 40 minutes.**
/ **Or – rest properly. Which is almost certainly what you need.**

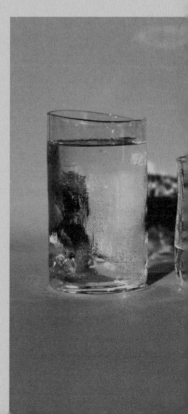

Hell is other people

All of that is fine if you're single and live alone. Clear out the booze, take your showers, do your crafts and don't look back. But there's a very good chance it's not that simple, and you do share your space with somebody who still drinks (or several who do). Of course it would be great if you could all leap on the wagon together and be each other's support buddies and laugh over board games while you sip elderflower cordial – but there's a high chance that ain't going to happen. So how can you manage giving up, or significantly cutting down, when your other half (or halves) is still drinking like Captain Jack Sparrow on a stag night?

A lot of online advice about this is apocalyptic. 'Tell them you WILL NOT put up with drunkenness', 'Find a sober partner', 'Move out', 'Insist that your housemates quit too'.

Er, you're the one that decided to give up, pal – you don't own the people around you. If you find you were only hanging out with them because you were drunk and mistakenly thought they were fun, that's different. But most of us have nurtured and cherished our close relationships for years, and although giving up booze is a big change, it doesn't mean everything else has to be upended – unless you want it to be.

The first thing to do is figure out how much you mind if people around you are drinking at home. If, at first, you're going to find it impossible to stare down the barrel of a bottle of pinot every night, you can ask – nicely – if your housemates can keep the booze away from you for a bit.

Maybe they could keep it in their rooms, say, or go out to a bar, or even join you in a non-alcoholic drink before dinner. But if your whole lives, up until now, have revolved around drink – Bloody Mary brunches, funny 'what I did last night OMG' discussions, shared hangovers watching rubbish Saturday morning TV, a big glass of wine while you discuss your day – it's going to be tough to change the mood at first. Again, we're back to 'change the routine'. And it's a good idea to plan in advance so that you can still function around the people you live with. Here's how…

Agree to move the booze / to break your habit.

Plan a regular 'nobody drinks' night / if they're up for it –
watching something slightly complex on Netflix is a good
idea for this.

If they're drinking half a bottle / (and you used to drink
the other half) buy a 35cl container and keep the half-bottle
of wine in that – this way, it's full and it's less mindlessly easy
to pour yourself a glass.

Stock up on 'pretend booze' / there is now a whole range
of alcohol-free wines, beers and distilled spirits available and
it really helps if you can pour yourself a glass of something
that at least looks like booze, rather then sipping a child's
party drink. It's also much cheaper than real booze – so keep
it on hand, and make sure you have ice. It may taste weird
at first, but it's an acquired taste, and after a month or so,
I acquired it. And you will too.

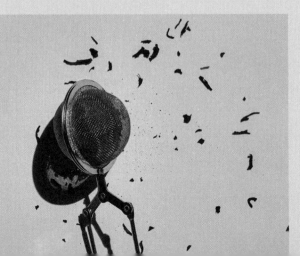

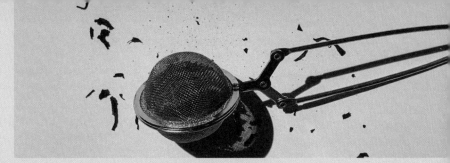

If you and your partner tend to unpack your day over a few drinks around the kitchen table or on the sofa, move the event / get in the bath and talk there, or sit in the garden (in summer, obviously; torturing yourself in minus seven just because you're sober would be demented).

Buy a huge variety of herbal teas to try / it will cost a few quid, but you thought nothing of spending a twenty on two bottles of store-bought prosecco in the past, and this will last a lot longer. It gives you an interesting taste to enjoy while your partner is chugging through another beer, and they're perfect for after dinner when you're watching TV and don't even notice what you're drinking anyway.

Remind them / I didn't particularly mind my partner saying 'glass of wine?' every night for the first three weeks, until he remembered I wasn't drinking – it gave me a slightly smug glow to know that I could refuse. But if you do mind (and why wouldn't you?), remind your co-habitee/s that you have decided not to drink, and it would be great if they could remember not to offer you alcohol, and not to try and persuade you to join them in drinking. It might feel slightly awkward at first, but what's more awkward than gathering with people purely so that you can absorb some flavoured ethanol into your bloodstream? Exactly.

The big rule / regarding housemates and partners, there is just one rule when you give up drinking…

Don't preach

Yes, you may well feel better, you may have seen the light, banished evil booze from your life and feel certain that if only your loved ones would do the same, you could all skip through rainbows down the yellow brick road to Paradise City.

This may be the case – but nobody likes an evangelist, and if they have chosen to drink, that's their 'journey' and it's up to them if or when they stop.

I asked my partner a few months in whether I'd changed since I gave up drinking. I was expecting 'Wow, yes, you're even more amazing', but he thought for a bit and said, 'You're a bit more… judge-y.'

Crushed and chastened, I realised he was right. I had turned into a booze-nag, forever pursing my lips when he poured another and murmuring, 'Are you sure you want to finish the bottle?' after dinner. I had mistaken my personal desire to stop drinking for a universal one.

Of course, if your partner has problems with alcohol, wants to stop but can't or becomes unpleasant when drunk, that's not about nagging – you have to decide whether to stick around and be supportive, or get the hell out.

And yes, it's annoying when your loved one is merrily making their way down a bottle of something on a Tuesday night, getting irritatingly tipsy, while you're stone-cold sober; again, you have the option of going to bed, reading a good book or just chatting back, marvelling like an anthropologist at how alcohol impacts the human brain.

The bottom line is, it's not your brain, it's theirs – and if they want to drink, they can. Don't ruin your good work by turning drinking into a good versus bad situation. It's a 'better for you at the moment' versus 'someone else's choice' situation – no matter how close you are.

However, that doesn't mean you can't tell them how great you feel without it.

Relationship corner

If your relationship was born in a club over shots, and developed over nights sharing wine, it's going to be difficult when one person takes their head out of the water (or vodka). It will change the dynamic of evenings in together – and that's something you should be aware of.

/ **You may find it harder to have deep, open conversations without drinking.**

/ **You might find you aren't laughing as much.**

/ **Plenty of couples are too shy to have sex without being mutually drunk, so how are you going to get naked sober?**

The obvious answer is, if it's a good relationship, it doesn't matter whether you're drunk or sober – you'll still want to talk, laugh and have sex. The less obvious answer is, it might take a bit of adjustment.

If you've grown accustomed to using 'being a bit pissed' as an excuse to open up, overcome your inhibitions and say what you really feel, not having that support can make you feel vulnerable, exposed and very shy. The balance between you will shift, particularly if your partner's still drinking. You might find…

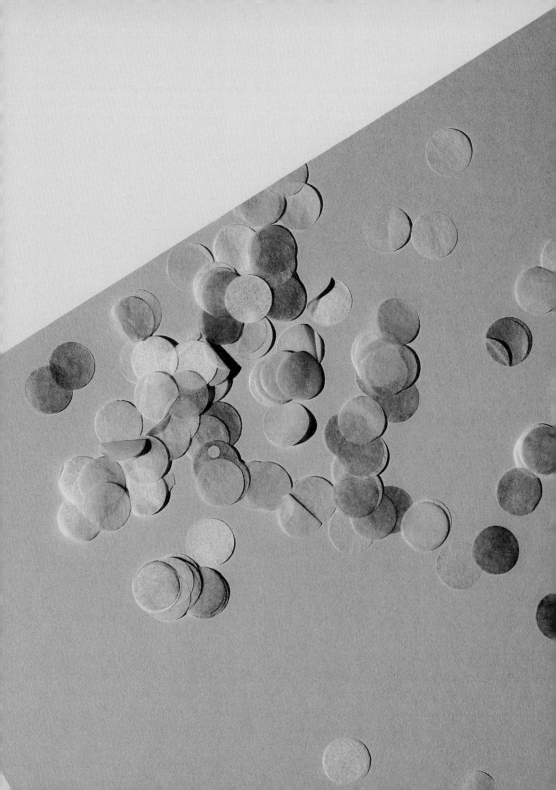

Your conversations aren't as instantly intense

Drink is a disinhibitor, which means it's easy to get from A to G (or even Z) in short order, bypassing B altogether. But it also means you're more emotional – and that means more likely to argue, to state feelings bluntly and to take offence more quickly. There is a big difference between intensity and intimacy – and drink often destroys the intimacy of genuine connection, while offering ramped-up emotional intensity in its place.

Save your serious conversations for when you're both sober, and if your partner is drinking – or drunk – keep things light. And if you can't? Go to bed. Emotional intensity is exhausting in other people too.

Your sex life is more awkward

Again, a few glasses of wine can certainly ease the path to fun, uninhibited sex, stripping away all the 'Is my stomach big? Do I look weird? Should I be noisier / quieter?' stuff along with your underwear. But again, true intimacy is best built sober, which is why you can have a wild one-night stand when you're drunk, but are barely able to look at one another sober at breakfast the next morning.

So yes, at first you may notice a little less confidence – but if you love your partner, you'll swiftly find that sex is actually better when you're not three sheets to the wind. And if you don't… it will give you the chance to assess whether you want to stick around without the booze.

If you're still drinking but cutting down

It can still be tricky to manage your intake when everyone around you is knocking it back like it's the night before battle. Here's how to do it...

Make a bottle of wine last almost a week / buy yourself one that only you will drink from – don't let anyone top you up from theirs. Go for a lower-alcohol white wine or rosé, as they will last up to a week in the fridge, and get a 125ml (4fl-oz) glass – one of those will mean it takes six days to finish, at a rate of one a day.

Buy a 25ml (1oz) measure / one of those equals one unit of spirits. Always use it when you make a mixer drink like G&T or whisky and soda. Otherwise it's very easy to do a 'home pour' and end up drinking triples without knowing it.

Buy a little glass for beer / and note the ABV on the bottle. For instance, Stella Artois is a whole lot more powerful that those tiny, fizzy French bottles.

Finally...

If you're staying in, reserve the right to leave any gathering and head for your room. You don't have to 'prove' to anyone that you're still fun without alcohol – all you have to do is not drink if you don't want to. So if you're tired, bored, irritated or craving a drink, go and get into bed, stick your headphones on and watch something distracting. You'll thank yourself in the morning.

Going
out

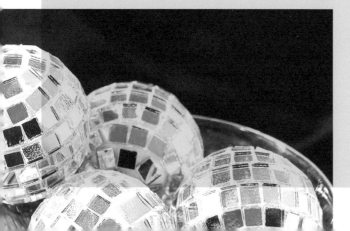

//

This is the masterclass of not drinking – the Rocky / Karate
Kid bit where you learn to be a better, stronger person
through denial and pain (though the pain is mostly caused
by other people, to be fair).

For anyone who drinks regularly, being out is the big trigger
– the lever in the brain that delivers the expected hit of fun,
the social life and off-the-leash, no-responsibility freedom.
Once pressed, it expects a dose of alcohol, and if you're out
– in a bar with the people you usually drink with, at a party
feeling nervous, waiting for a Tinder date or at a wedding
where you don't know anyone – your conditioned brain
is automatically ready and waiting for that numbing shot
of ethanol.

And when it doesn't arrive, there's a lot less distraction
and avoidance available than there is at home. Basically,
everything is the same, everyone is the same (still drinking);
the only difference is you, you're not drinking. So here's
how to cope…

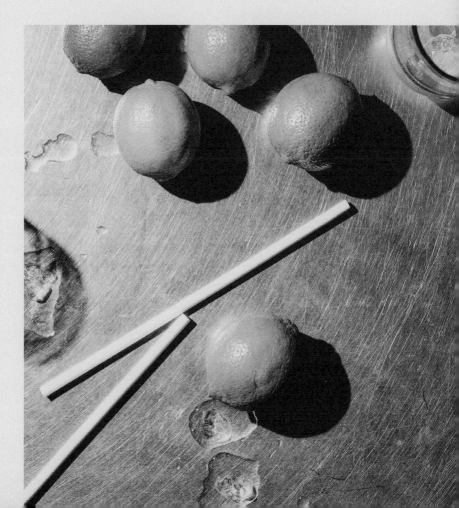

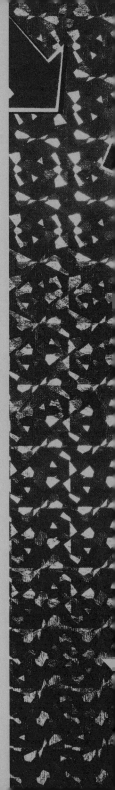

Have an exit plan

Those old drunken evenings that rolled on through weird chats with strangers, wandering off to a party, losing an hour two and finding yourself on the night bus clutching a McDonald's, are over – for now, at least. And getting caught up in someone else's unmapped choose-your-own-adventure Friday night when you're on the Diet Coke is not fun. So the first thing you need, before the evening even starts, is an exit strategy. That way, you know how you're getting home, and if it all gets too much (by 10pm everyone has their arms round each other and they're singing football songs), you can gracefully leave, without having to worry about how. Make sure you do one of the following…

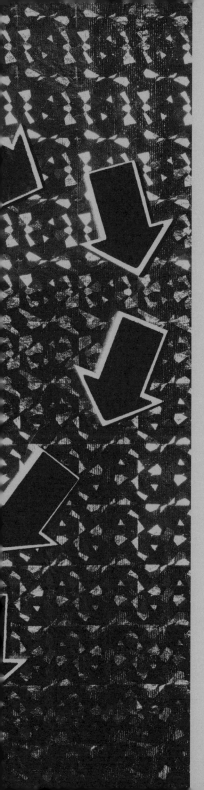

Check the train or bus times / and decide
which one you'll get – and what time you'll therefore have
to go.

Arrange a lift / your partner, friend or whoever will
be outside the venue at a certain time, and that's when you
need to go.

Order a cab in advance / and make sure you're
waiting outside.

It may seem a good idea to be the designated driver, but
that will mean you're left hanging on while the bell for last
orders goes and your drunken friends are still shrieking with
laughter and shouting, 'One more drink, then we're coming!'

Be selfish at first; do what you need to do, and that means
leaving yourself an exit route, so if temptation strikes – or
you just realise that without booze you're knackered by
9.30pm – you can quietly leave.

To tell or not to tell?

The first few times you go out sober, let your friends or dates know when you plan to leave – and though they will plead, 'Nooo, stay!', just say that you can't because you have to be up early. Or tell the truth – that you really want to see them, but might struggle later, once the booze kicks in.

That way you won't get a chorus of drunken disappointment and pestering when you say 'Bye' later on. (Or you will, and can just say, 'I told you I was leaving early'.)

But on certain occasions, and depending on who you are with, you may not want to announce to the world that you've given up drinking, mainly because it's your decision, and declaring it publicly is a full-scale invitation to comment. Likely responses include…

'Forever?!'

'Oh, come on. Just cut down if you're worried.'

'What are you on about, it's not like you're an alcoholic!'

'I drink more than you do, don't be ridiculous.'

'Oh, thanks. Who will I go out with now, then?'

'Tell me you're not giving up until after the wedding / big night / mini-break...'

'Look, I've bought you one now, so you may as well drink it and start again tomorrow.'

'Oh great, the Fun Police are in town.'

'Just have a beer then.'

'Seriously? But you're the biggest drinker I know!'

'Whaaat? Are you in AA?'

'WHY?'

And many, many variations on the above.

Your nearest and dearest may have been privy to your inner wranglings about whether or not to quit, and may (or may not) be fully in support. But your booze friends, your workmates, your friends-of-friends – they may well be startled by your (to them) sudden decision. When you tell them what you've decided, it could go any number of ways; here are some probable scenarios…

They will want to reassure you / ('You don't drink much anyway!'), in the hope that you'll return to normal, feeling better about yourself, and can drink along with them again.

They will ignore you / by buying you a drink anyway, or pouring you a glass, they will override what they see as your feeble objections and just assume you don't really mean it.

They will mock you / by undermining your intention not to drink, making jokes and laughing at your 'boring' choice, they hope you'll give in and rejoin the drinkers, rather than risk being cast out of your tribe.

They will be annoyed / usually only if they're drunk themselves. But there's a good chance at least one will decide that what you need is a heated debate, focusing intently on why you're wrong not to drink. And they won't give up until you're necking a giant glass of wine or a pint of lager.

So why is it so difficult to simply say, 'I'm not drinking', and have everyone else say, 'OK!'?

There are several reasons. Chiefly, nobody likes it when an accepted member of the tribe suddenly differentiates themselves. It's primal and basic, because the pack is weakened when you aren't all acting as one.

But a further compelling reason is that, deep down, they fear your decision means bad things.

That the fun will stop / because the consensus is that drinking is good, it's what you all do together and that's great; the fear is that things may fall apart if someone doesn't go along with it.

That maybe you do all drink too much / and if you quit, that means they might have to look at their own drinking; they don't want to and will resent you for shining a spotlight on their own uncomfortable feelings.

They see it as an abandonment and betrayal of your friendship / if it's been largely based on co-drinking, you appear to be saying, 'I'm out'; it feels like a rejection of your shared time and values.

You know that none of these things are true (unless they are, in which case your choice of friendship group might need a rethink, and that's fair enough), but drinking is a far more emotive issue than it first appears, woven through friendships, intimacy, sex and socialising. Which is why, with those people you suspect will give you grief of any sort, it can make sense to lie – particularly if you don't see them often. You can't keep on lying if you see them every week and you're always clutching an orange juice, but if you just need to get through the evening without temptation and hassle, try the following messages of the truth…

When they say, 'What are you drinking?' / just say, 'Oh, I'm not doing rounds, I get out of sync, so don't worry.' If they are annoyingly insistent, tell them you're driving.

Say you're driving / (or actually drive). And if they say, 'Oh, you can have a couple', say you had one before you came out. Just to shut them up.

Use the old antibiotics excuse / very few people are rude enough to ask, 'What for?'

Try saying you're having a night off / (though this leaves you open to persuasion and nagging).

Big day tomorrow, up at the crack of dawn – can't risk a hangover / (you may then need to invent a big day, so be careful with this one).

The actual drink lie / drink sparkling water with lime, in a G&T glass. And make sure you're not near anyone else when you order. Be wary of anyone asking, 'Can I have a sip?', though.

Overall, it's simpler to tell the truth, but if you think a white lie will make your life easier at first, do it with conviction.

The types of night out

Not all nights out are the same, so here are some ways to handle different situations:

Date

In theory, this should be the easiest night out to navigate booze free. But that very much depends whether it's with a long-term partner (who we'll assume will already know) or someone you've exchanged three mildly flirtatious Tinder messages with.

It's not that they have any right to tell you whether to drink or not – simply that without the false confidence generated by a shared bottle, the conversation may never quite get going. Or if they are ploughing on alone, it may take off in an entirely unexpected direction. It may be tempting to give in and 'just have a couple' to be polite. Which may well turn into a bottle. So avoid the whole tricky scenario in advance by mentioning that you're not drinking; if they ask, 'Why not?', remind yourself that you don't owe them an explanation. A simple 'I just feel better without it for now' should be enough. And if they try to persuade you? That's a red flag for 'thinks they know best, doesn't listen'. Which is useful when it comes to deciding on a second date.

Work drinks

In many ways, this is the big nightmare. Celebrating someone's promotion, an end-of-the-week moan, a team-bonding trip to the local bar… they all require alcohol. And because you don't really know Beth from HR and Sanjeet from Systems, the only way the less-than-wildly-extroverted person can traditionally cope with these 'forced fun' occasions is by drinking alcohol, to aid the dry-as-dust small talk, or to make the ironic karaoke session bearable, depending on your type of workplace. Without it, the evening yawns ahead.

Initially, while you're still likely to be tempted to drink, the best solution is to avoid it altogether. Invent a cousin you're picking up from the airport or similar. If you can't avoid it altogether, though, the best approach is 'intense but brief'. Commit yourself to talking to at least five different people, show great interest in their thoughts and achievements and make your presence noted – then leave, after max two hours.

If you can't leave, and they're all drunk, remind yourself that without drink you will never risk losing your job by a) saying something stupid while drunk, or b) turning up to work so hungover that you can't function. Your colleagues, of course, will run that risk.

And if your boss buys you a drink and it's too awkward to say, 'No, thanks', just accept then take it to the bathroom with you and pour it away. And before you say, 'But it's a waste…', remember that's it's just cheap, toxic ethanol – better down the sink than through your liver and bladder, isn't it?

Catch-up with friends

Ideally, when you see friends, they'll already know you're not drinking. But if you haven't seen them for a while, they'll probably assume you're still the fun hell-raiser you were at university, and may have got the drinks in before you arrived. There's nothing like a reunion to make people want to drink – initially to overcome the awkwardness of meeting again, and then to fuel the hilarious recollections and cover up the fact that maybe you don't have that much in common any more.

But once you've practised saying, 'I'm not drinking at the moment, but it's no big deal – I'll just nip to the bar', and returned with your G&T-lookalike lime and soda, the conversation will have moved on.

Be straightforward, be casual about it and don't appear to be judging their choices – there's no reason for it to ruin anyone's evening.

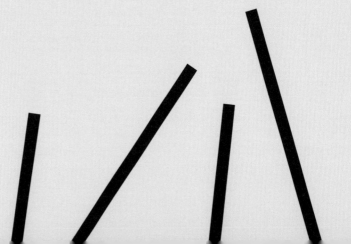

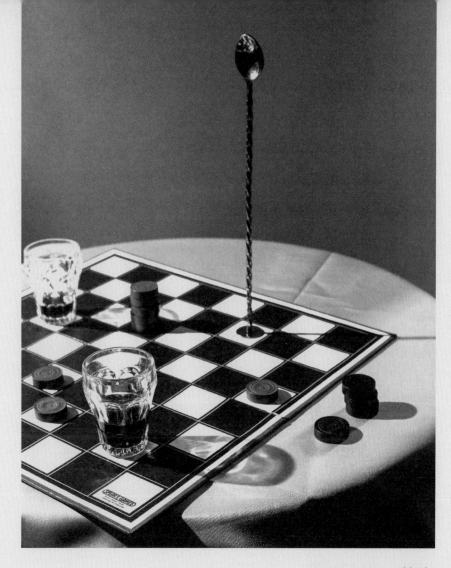

Note: A woman suddenly 'not drinking' can lead to all kinds of unnecessary rumours about pregnancy. Nip them in the bud.

Quitting the habit

Not the booze habit – you've already done that. (I don't believe that giving up booze is a lifelong process of 'recommitting every day' and so on – it can be if you're an alcoholic, but for many of us, it's a simple matter of making one important decision and sticking to it. It's like being faithful to your partner – you may be tempted to stray, but a quick mental run-through of the consequences, and you know it's not worth it. Unless it is, but that's when the metaphor falls apart.)

The habits you need to quit – or rather the ones you need to change – are your going-out habits, because once again, the human brain works on simple, idiot-friendly tracks. And if you do something a lot, your basic brain will assume you're going to keep doing it, and get you all primed and ready – particularly when it comes to addictive substances like alcohol.

So if you always go for a drink with your friends on a Friday evening, as you pack up after work, your brain will already be painting that cartoon picture of a shining glass filled with lovely, thirst-quenching beer; if you meet your best friend for dinner every fortnight and you always drink the same pinot, there your brain goes, ready and waiting for cold white wine even as you get in the cab. Which is why it's a great idea to do something different that doesn't automatically trigger 'drinking' thoughts, but still allows you to have a social life and go out.

Here are a few ideas to try that won't make life hard for your friends or for you...

Instead of: Meeting for cocktails.

Try: Meeting for brunch. That way, your friends can have bottomless prosecco or Bloody Marys and you can have coffee and orange juice. There isn't the same pressure to drink at noon, strangely enough.

Instead of: Going for a fancy dinner date.

Try: Going for a fancy picnic, which also means you'll probably drive. (Note: Don't do this with someone you barely know. Go for coffee.)

Instead of: Meeting the boys for a beer.

Try: A game of five-a-side. They might all head off for a beer afterwards of course, but by then, your drinking-urge-associated-with-leaving-work will have ebbed.

Instead of: A girls' night out.

Try: A girls' day out – take a dance class, go to a theme park, have afternoon tea somewhere posh.

At first, all this takes a bit of extra planning – and possibly persuasion – but once the neural pathway with its big 'Alcohol this way' sign is weakened, it won't be as hard to go to a bar and order Diet Coke without wincing in pain. Talking of which...

What to drink out when you're not drinking

In the past, there were roughly five choices in the average bar or pub. Orange juice, in a little sticky bottle, tonic water, Coke / Diet Coke (or Pepsi) or soda water, possibly with lime if you were feeling exotic. Occasionally, a generous landlord would invest in some pineapple juice or Appletiser, and if you were really glam you could have a St Clements – bitter lemon mixed with orange juice. Or perhaps a shandy – because as all dads know, lager mixed with lemonade magically becomes non-alcoholic, and allows you to drive anywhere afterwards. (Note: This is not true.)

Basically it was grim, and although this is still pretty much the offering in some traditional 'what are you doing here if you don't want a pint and a white wine for the lady' drinking establishments, most places have moved on a bit. There is a vast array of possibilities for the sober and sober-curious, and if your local doesn't stock them, keep asking – because the bigger the demand, the more likely they are to bother. Some drinks, such as Seedlip and Ceder – non-alcoholic distilled spirits – are now served in more high-end bars and restaurants, many have the Fentimans range of rediscovered 'Victorian' classics and sophisticated Fever-Tree tonics, but even the most spit-and-sawdust joints will at least offer J2O and Britvic.

Here are some options to look for that won't mean you feel like a five-year-old with your half pint of draught lemonade all night, and which won't pump you with enough sugar to trigger a diabetic coma.

1 Elderflower fizz / and grapefruit juice over ice. Yes, you will have to pay for two mini bottles – but it's still cheaper than a pint, and offers a hit of pleasing sharpness.

2 Soda water with Angostura bitters / and a dash of lime. Bitters are alcoholic, but it's such a tiny amount that it doesn't count.

3 Virgin Mary / the whole tomato juice, Worcestershire sauce and Tabasco thing, without the vodka. Make it spicy enough to drink slowly.

4 Cranberry and lime / topped with soda. Refreshing, and good for your urinary tract, fact fans.

5 Non-alcoholic beer / tastes not that far off the real thing – BrewDog and Beck's Blue are easy to drink and ensure you don't stand out from the crowd.

6 Non-alcoholic wine / many bars are very far behind the curve when it comes to stocking alcohol-free wines like Eisberg, but there's no harm asking.

7 Ginger beer / 'Victorian' fizzes / the 'traditional' types such as Fentimans are much more interesting than the standard mixers. See also their Dandelion & Burdock, Curiousity Cola and Rose Lemonade – all more sophisticated tastes than the kiddy equivalent.

8 Shirley Temple / ginger beer with grenadine over ice – a bit of a kick and a fun novelty. But don't drink them all night, or you'll feel as queasy as if you'd drunk ten Pornstar Martinis.

9 Diet Coke / Coke and its similar alternatives. This is the obvious one to order. But half pint after half pint of Coke becomes insanely dull and heavy on the bladder, so try a half and half of Diet Coke and cranberry juice for a longer, more interesting drink.

10 Sparkling water / with a slice of lime. Sounds dull, but you'll feel great at the end of the night, as it's sugar free, hydrating and every bar will serve it. Add a dash of Angostura bitters to liven it up if the staff don't mind.

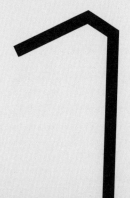

Three magical* ways to stay sober when out

1 **Borrow a trick from therapy /** make a list of all the things you love about being sober, then memorise it while you ping an elastic band on your wrist, or rub a pendant – any ritual you can do discreetly while you're out. If cravings strike, perform your little ritual to be instantly reminded of why you're not drinking.

2 **Use an app /** sites like Club Soda and Soberistas are packed with tips and advice for resisting temptation. Keep them on your phone, and if you're wavering, scroll through for a boost – everyone will assume you're just checking Instagram or Snapchat.

3 **Enlist a sober buddy /** who you can talk to when everyone else is getting hammered. Ideally, they'll be another designated driver, or non-boozer. If they're not with you in person, arrange to message them every so often with an update and get a swift line or two of support in return. If no such person exists, once the slurring and singing starts, it's probably time to make your excuses and leave.

*Not actually magical; please don't sue me.

What to drink instead

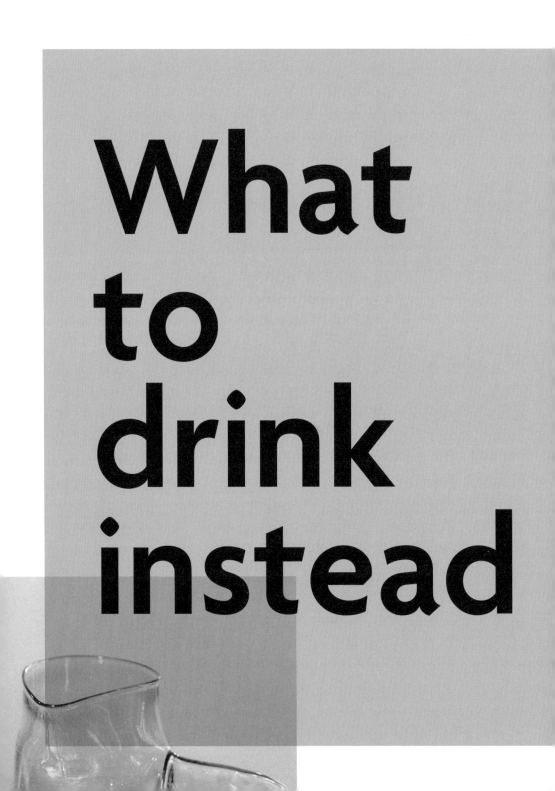

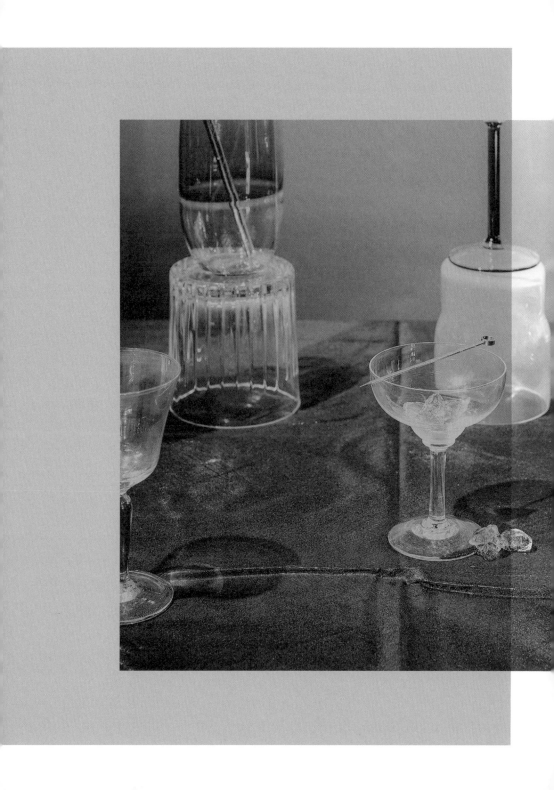

The mocktails served in restaurants and bars are often 90 per cent syrup and soda. They're a brutal approximation of the real thing – a cheap splash of sherbet-flavoured soft drink, ice and a slice of strawberry, costing nearly as much as a double whisky. Some bars' offerings are far better than this, of course, and will go out of their way to make you something that doesn't taste like a liquidised party bag from a five-year-old's birthday – but really great mocktails are still in their infancy. So for now, the best place to make and drink them is at home, a place where you can take your time to mix them properly, and drink them in good company.

Certain cocktails – primarily gin- or champagne-based ones – lend themselves to alcohol-free replication, thanks to the joys of Seedlip or Ceder non-alcoholic distilled spirits and non-alcoholic prosecco. But there are plenty of others that may not taste quite like whisky, say, but certainly capture a sense of that peaty, smoky richness, or conjure up the zingy kick of vodka. Not everyone wants their mocktail to taste like alcohol – some prefer a fruity or refreshing taste. But all these recipes look and taste like something a discerning adult would enjoy, rather than something so full of sugar that it will trigger a toddler tantrum before bed.

Build a mocktail cabinet

If you're going to do it properly, you need the right tools.
If you don't already own them, invest in the following:

/ Cocktail shaker

/ Muddler

/ Strainer

/ Jigger (measure)

/ Small whisk

/ Small, sharp knife

/ Peeler

/ Lighter

/ Set of measuring spoons

/ Selection of glasses,
    including tumblers,
    coupes, martini glasses
    and highball glasses*

*And if you also have a 1950s mirrored cocktail cabinet, so much the better.

Next, you need to stock up on some useful ingredients so that you've always got something you can turn into a delicious mocktail:

/ **Non-alcoholic distilled spirits**

/ **Non-alcoholic wine and prosecco**

/ **Cassis (blackcurrant) syrup**

/ **Caramel syrup**

/ **Limonata**

/ **Grenadine syrup**

/ **Maraschino cherries**

/ **Stem ginger in syrup**

/ **Sparkling water or soda water**

/ **Fruit juices, including apple, tomato, orange and cranberry**

/ **Elderflower cordial**

/ **Citrus fruits, including lemons, limes and satsumas**

/ **Berries**

/ **Ice**

Note: The following mocktails will work without the non-alcoholic distilled spirit, but they won't taste as close to the real thing. That, however, may not be a bad thing.

All recipes serve 1.

Manhattan

This is a very sophisticated drink, for those times you want to feel you're in a panelled apartment in old New York, sitting in front of a crackling fire, talking about Bunty and Chet heading to the Hamptons in spring.

1 maraschino cocktail cherry; plus 1 to decorate

½ tsp caramel syrup (Monin is good)

45ml / 3 tbsp non-alcoholic distilled spirit

¼ tsp grenadine syrup

45ml / 3 tbsp non-alcoholic red wine

¼ tsp syrup from the maraschino cocktail cherry jar

2 drops Angostura bitters (these are alcoholic but barely in such small amounts. Replace with non-alcoholic bitters if preferred)

4 large ice cubes

Put one cherry into the bottom of a champagne coupe or whisky tumbler.

Pour all the other ingredients into a cocktail shaker with the ice cubes. Shake vigorously for around a minute.

Check it's cold, then strain the mix into the glass. Decoarte with the extra cherry threaded onto a cocktail stick. Sip, and eat the cherries afterwards.

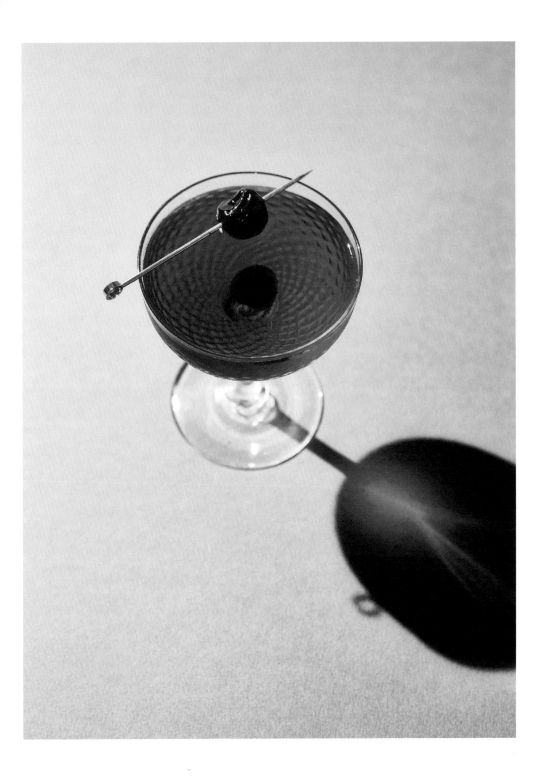

Piña colada

ice cubes
150ml / 5fl oz pineapple juice
1 tsp caramel syrup
50ml / 2fl oz coconut water
50ml / 2fl oz coconut cream
   (the thick part of
   an unshaken can
   of coconut milk)
juice of ½ lime
slice of pineapple

Perfect if you like getting caught in the rain, you're not much into yoga and you have half a brain. This tropical drink conjures up beaches, breezes and fun.

Fill a cocktail shaker with ice.

Add all the other ingredients except the pineapple slice. Shake vigorously for at least a minute.

Strain slowly into a large balloon glass and add the slice of pineapple to the rim.

Pornstar martini

2 ice cubes

2 tsp passion fruit syrup
  (or use the flesh of
  1 fresh passion fruit
  and 1 tsp sugar syrup)

25ml / 1fl oz non-alcoholic
  distilled spirit

1 tsp lime juice

2 drops natural vanilla extract

non-alcoholic prosecco, to
  top up

**This slightly less than classy-sounding drink was only
invented in 2002, but it tastes so great we can overlook
the name. This mocktail is very easy to drink – but be
warned, it contains a lot of sugar.**

Add the ice cubes to a cocktail shaker.

If you are using fresh passion fruit, muddle it in the shaker
before adding the sugar syrup, non-alcoholic spirit, lime
juice and vanilla extract. If not, just add all ingredients
except the prosecco to the shaker.

Shake vigorously until mixed and strain into a martini glass.
Top up to just below the rim with the 'prosecco'.

Old fashioned

ice cubes

strip of lemon peel, pith removed

50ml / 2fl oz non-alcoholic distilled spirit

½ tsp caramel syrup

2 drops Angostura bitters (or use non-alcoholic bitters)

This is a remarkably delicious, alcohol-free version of a simple whisky cocktail, to be drunk in stately homes at Christmas, as you squabble over the inheritance. (Or in your living room, watching TV – it works either way.)

Half-fill a whisky tumbler with ice.

On a hard surface, gently bash the lemon peel with a muddler to release the oil.

Pour the remaining ingredients into the glass, add the strip of lemon peel and stir.

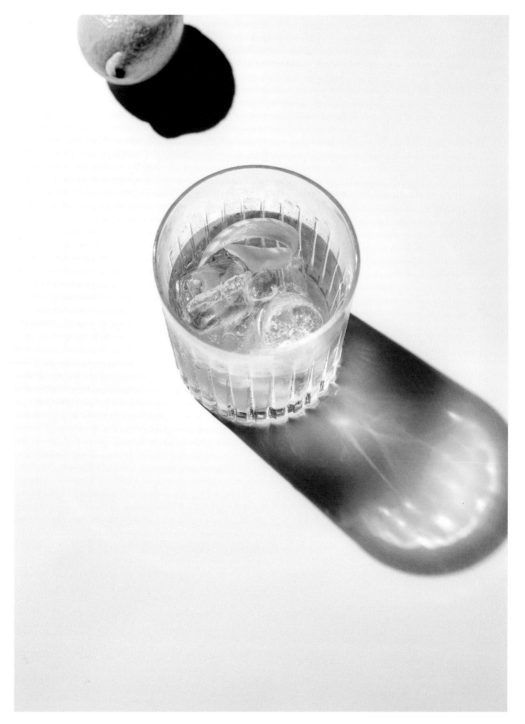

Dark invader

3–4 ice cubes
6 blueberries
50ml / 2fl oz pineapple juice
25ml / 1fl oz sugar syrup
25ml / 1fl oz plain water
½ tsp cassis syrup
strip of lemon peel, pith
    removed
can of San Pellegrino
    Limonata

This is a grown-up, fruity cocktail that is perfect on a summer evening in the garden, or just as good in autumn, as you watch the rain fall outside. It's mature, without being bitter.

Put the ice cubes into a short tumbler. Put the blueberries into a cocktail shaker and muddle until they are broken up.

Add the pineapple juice, sugar syrup, water and cassis syrup to the shaker. Shake and strain into a glass.

Use a muddler to lightly bash the lemon peel and add it to the glass.

Top up the glass to just below rim with the San Pellegrino Limonata. Stir.

Forest fruits daiquiri

5 blackberries, plus 1
   to decorate
5 raspberries
ice cubes
½ tsp raspberry syrup
¼ tsp caramel syrup
50ml / 2fl oz non-alcoholic
   distilled spirit (optional)
juice of ½ lime

The Daiquiri is the 'Well, hello, Mr Bond' of cocktails. This booze-free version still packs a lovely punch, and can be sipped elegantly overlooking Hong Kong harbour from a 99th floor suite – or served at a small mocktail soirée in your basement flat.

Put the berries into a cocktail shaker and bash with a muddler until the juice is released.

Add ice to the shaker, followed by the remaining ingredients. Shake vigorously.

Strain through a fine mesh into a martini glass and decorate with a blackberry.

Mojito

a handful of fresh mint,
   stalks removed
ice cubes
½ tsp caramel syrup
½ tsp sugar syrup
50ml / 2fl oz non-alcoholic
   distilled spirit
juice of ½ lime
sparkling water or soda
   water; to top up

**This classic cocktail can very easily taste of nothing if
you don't get the quantities right. Done well, you're in a
Copacabana beach bar, laughing with close friends. Done
badly, you're in your kitchen, grimly sipping mouthwash.
This one, however, gets pretty close to the real thing.**

Put the mint leaves into a tall glass, reserving a small sprig to
decorate. Use a muddler to lightly bash the leaves until they
are broken up and smelling highly minty.

Fill the glass to the top with ice cubes. Pour in the rest of
the ingredients except the sparkling / soda water and stir.

Top up to taste with sparkling / soda water and decorate
with the reserved sprig of mint.

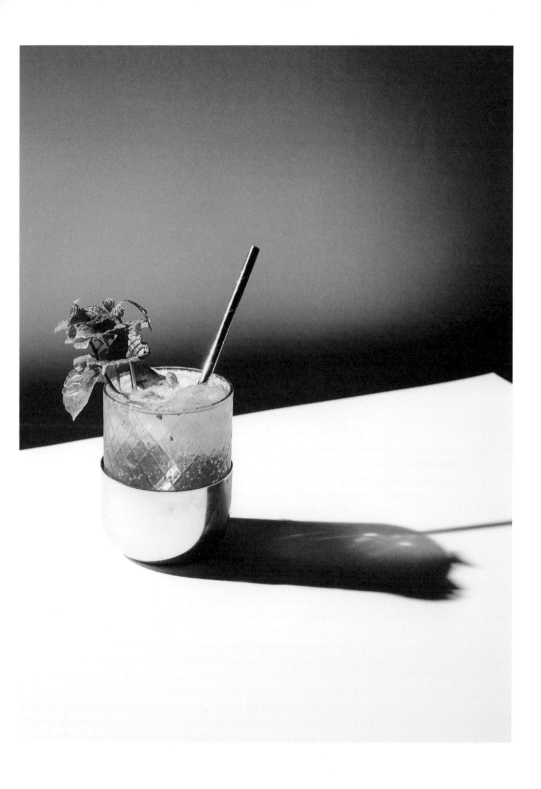

Cosmopolitan

½ satsuma, peeled and
   segmented
ice cubes
30ml / 2 tbsp cranberry juice
10ml / 2 tsp lime juice
¼ tsp sugar syrup
strip of orange peel,
   pith removed

Sex and the City is long over – and its legacy of
unaffordable NYC apartments, terrible innuendo and
obsessing over awful men has gone too. But there is one
iconic memory that the show left behind – the Cosmo.
The drink equivalent of a gentle kick from a Manolo
Blahnik. It also works without alcohol (and invariably
leads to better relationship choices).

Put the satsuma segments into a cocktail shaker and use a
muddler to lightly bash them until all the juice is released.
Add a handful of ice cubes, followed by all the remaining
ingredients except the orange peel.

Shake vigorously, then strain into a martini glass.

Bend the strip of orange peel over the glass. Using a lighter,
gently run a flame over the outer surface of the peel to
release the oil.

Cucumberbatch

½ cucumber
ice cubes
50ml / 2fl oz non-alcoholic
    distilled spirit (I like
    Seedlip here)
50ml / 2fl oz sparkling
    elderflower drink

**This gloriously simple cocktail is summer in a glass.
There's a bit of faff required to juice the cucumber –
you will need a juicer, or you can peel, blend and strain
the juice through a sieve. You can do a couple at once
and save it for the next day.**

First, juice the cucumber in a juicer (or peel and blend in
a food processor or blender) then strain. Put a handful of
ice cubes into a cocktail shaker.

Add 75ml / 5 tbsp of the cucumber juice and the
non-alcoholic distilled spirit. Shake vigorously.

Strain into a martini glass and top up with the sparkling
elderflower drink.

Virgin Mary

3–4 ice cubes
110ml / 4fl oz tomato juice
5ml / 1 tsp Worcestershire
   sauce
5ml / 1 tsp lemon juice
1 tsp horseradish
   (creamed from a jar
   is fine, but fresh would
   be best if you can get
   hold of it)
1–3 drops Tabasco sauce
sprinkle of celery salt
black pepper
celery stick, to garnish

This is a stormer of a breakfast cocktail to wake you up – you don't really need the vodka at all. Drink in crisp cotton pyjamas sitting on a balcony with your new love. Or in bed alone with the cat and the papers.

Put the ice cubes into a highball glass.

Add all the other ingredients to taste – start with just 1 drop of Tabasco and add more if you want it very spicy.

Stir and add the celery stick.

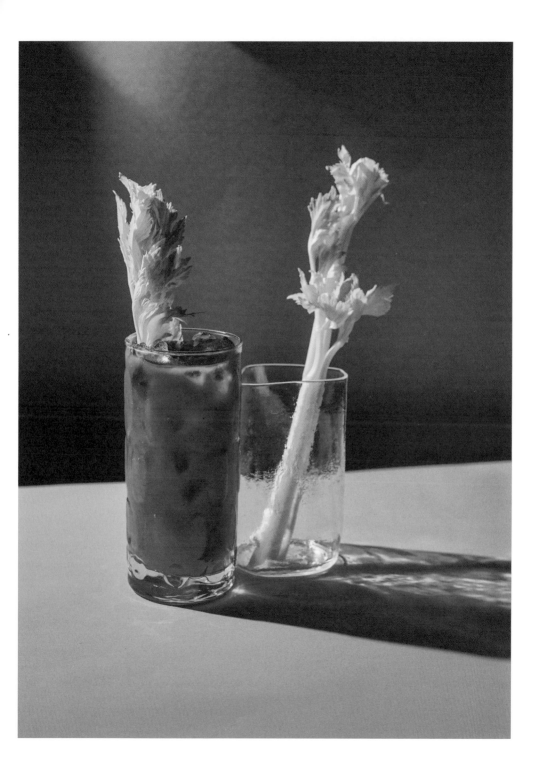

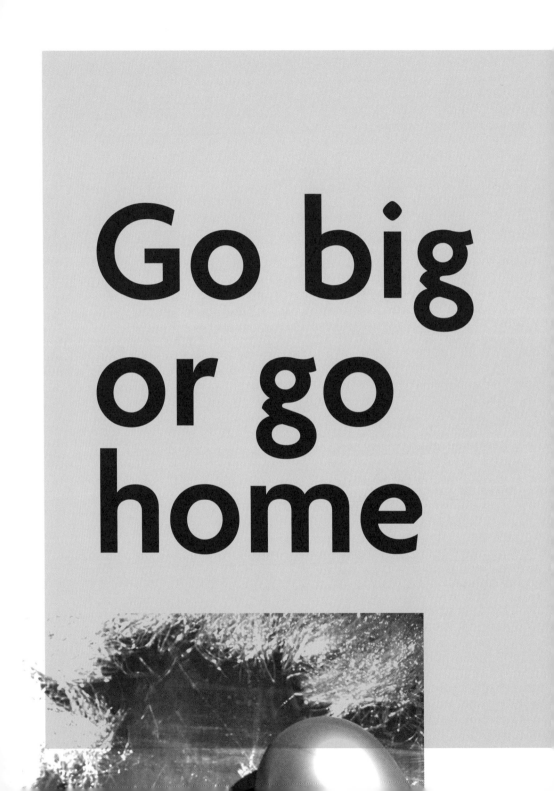

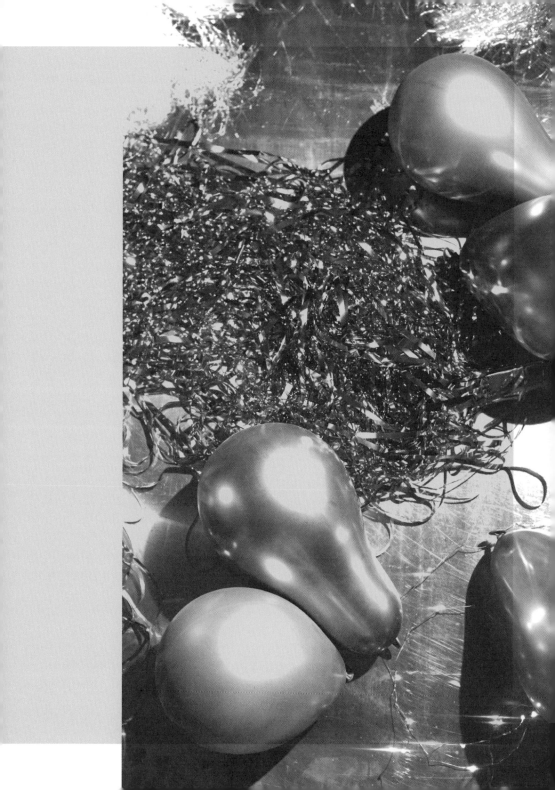

This is the final frontier of not drinking – The Event. Culturally, most of us are used to boozing whenever something major happens, much like being trapped in a lifelong drinking game. Christmas: Drink! Birthday: Drink! Wedding: Drink! Funeral: Oh God, yes, drink! From New Year to vacations to friends' Big Birthdays (there's always someone having a Big Birthday), it's almost impossible to dodge through life, Frogger-like, without someone thrusting a glass into your hand and shouting 'Cheers!'

But when you want to celebrate yet don't want to end
the joyous evening by swaying and crying in front of the
mirror (or worse), how do you navigate the situation? You
may have mastered the art of sitting quietly in a bar or pub
nursing a lime and soda, but sipping water to toast the bride
and groom or avoiding the popping corks at midnight as
another year begins is another level of sober altogether. It's
very likely you'll be the only straight-edge person in the
room, and big events also tend to mean that you can't just
slope off, unnoticed, if it all gets a bit much. But I promise it
can be done – and you'll even enjoy yourself. Honest.

How to approach big events

The first thing to do is change your expectations. We've been conditioned to associate celebratory drinking with having fun – and if 'wedding' has always meant 'getting wasted with old friends, hitting the dance floor like Beyoncé and kissing someone inappropriate', it's going to be tough without the tasty chemical that enabled all that. Equally, if New Year means 'we always see the same close friends and get hammered on champagne and play hilarious drunken games', approaching the evening sober can feel a lot like turning up to a festival in a business suit. There's also the element of big events that involves small talk with strangers (always easier after a few glasses of champagne) and the fact that they tend to go on for hours, so without drinking, you'll not only feel the odd one out, you'll also be out of your mind with boredom.

These are all valid concerns – I had them myself. But having now managed all of the Big Events sober, I'm here to tell you it's not that difficult at all – you simply have to view them differently.

Your past self believed that helping a friend celebrate, marking some major life stage of your own or celebrating Father Christmas having turned up meant drinking enough alcohol to destroy all your inhibitions, throwing yourself into partying and waking up with a hangover and a very hazy recall of anything that happened after 10pm.

However, your current (sober) self needs to look at the situation with a fresh pair of eyes.

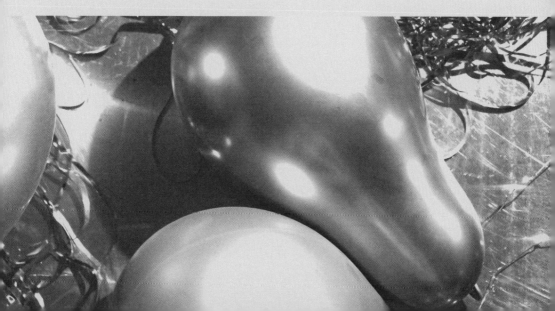

These big events are most often situations that are really important to you, your friends or your family (or all three). They need to go smoothly, and your role is to help that happen by being fun, sociable, pleasant and helpful when required.

Your friends did not say, 'I know, let's get married so our friend can get smashed at our expense.' / they want you there because they like you and hope you being there will enhance their day, and that you will also have a good time.

Your family did not book a luxury weekend away for Dad's 70th / so you could crack open the wine every night and get up at noon with a blazing hangover that makes you irritable and unhelpful until cocktail hour.

Your kids did not spend eight weeks preparing for Christmas Day with wild excitement / so you could sit glumly through the present-opening, waiting for your chance to start drinking.

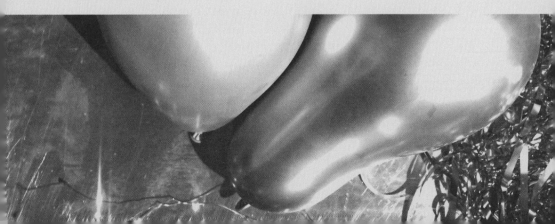

Your friends didn't bring champagne for New Year because they think you'll be no fun without it / they brought it because it's traditional and they hoped you'd all have a glass. It doesn't mean you need to be so trolleyed by midnight that you can barely see to pour it out.

You did not invite loads of people to your 30th (or 21st, or 50th) / so you could sink a crate of booze, embarrass yourself flirting with the wrong person and forget most of the night.

Basically, your fundamental role at events is to join in with the fun, not to join in with the drinking. You'll have perfect recall, dance without falling over and wake up for the massive hotel breakfast without a hangover.

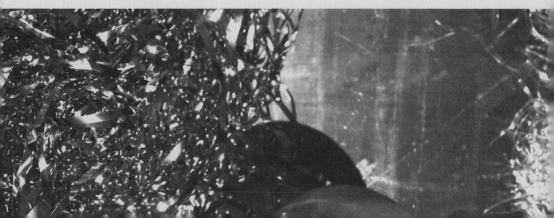

Here's how to manage The Big Ones, clean, sober and having fun. (Apart from the funeral.)

Weddings

From the first glass of champagne (or cava from the French hypermarket) at the reception, to the wine with the wedding meal, to the toasts, to the brandies (or beers) in the bar later, weddings are a sea of alcohol. They also tend to last for at least ten hours, which means a full day of drinking, while the only way to avoid a crippling hangover kicking in around 5pm is simply to keep on drinking. So don't begin. Not one glass of 'celebratory' champagne, not one just-a-red-wine-with-the-beef, not a single 'toasting the bride so it doesn't really count' sip of fizz.

Because if you do, it will be very hard to stop – once you're holding a glass, waiters will feel duty bound to fill it up, your throat will be dry from talking to old friends and random aunties, and you'll keep drinking and the glass will keep filling. And at that point, you'll be tipsy enough to forget all your resolutions about how you're not going to drink much.

So make a solemn vow to yourself that you won't have the first one, and steam straight in with the canapés.

If there's orange juice offered, have one to show willing, then move on to whatever non-alcoholic alternatives are on offer. I suggest a hip flask containing ginger or elderflower cordial to cheer up your sparkling mineral water – a quick dash when nobody's looking will work wonders. (If they are looking, they'll assume you're a cheapskate adding vodka, but then, you'll never have to see them again…)

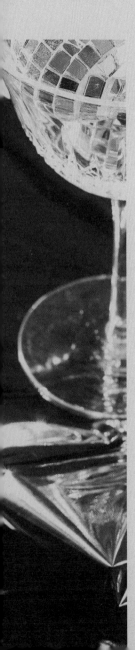

Tackling shyness

There's no bigger small-talk-with-strangers opportunity than at a wedding, and if you're socially shy, it's a challenge without a boost of false confidence. The fact is, though, if you feel sick at the thought of mingling, you don't have to. Drift over to the terrace and admire the lawn, or drift over to the walls and admire the local council notices, depending on what type of wedding it is. There's a good chance someone will talk to you, and if they do, all you have to do is answer their polite questions, and ask a few back. One might well be, 'Aren't you drinking?', which will almost certainly lead to quite an interesting conversation about why not, and how they really think they should stop too. At the sit-down bit, wine will be poured – make sure there's water or a soft drink near you so that you can pour your own. Discreetly asking a waiter should sort it – and again, let others kick off the talking, and join in only when you need to.

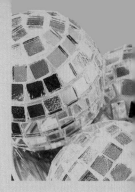

Toasting

Champagne will be poured for the toast. You can either wave it away and toast with your water glass, or you can simply lift the glass without drinking. It will not magically curse the happy couple if a random guest doesn't swallow a mouthful of Moët, trust me.

Making speeches

OK, this is trickier. Most of us are terrified of public speaking, and if it's your job to do so, it's natural to want to take the edge off the terror with a glass of something first. However, of all the (many) weddings you have to attend, the worst are those with a drunk best man (or woman). Everyone cringes in horror as he or she stumbles through rambling anecdotes and mistimed jokes, and claps violently when it's over out of sheer relief.

You might think you can have just one drink to steady your nerves and still be brilliant – you can't. This is a speech the couple will remember forever. Everyone will forgive a few nerves and stammers on such a big occasion. Few will forgive a best man selfish enough to make it all about him. Deal with nerves by taking a few long, deep breaths and a drink of water, and reminding yourself that everyone wants to laugh, and if they don't, it doesn't matter anyway. What matters is that you honour your friends properly.

Dancing

By the time the dancing starts, most people are pretty drunk. It's admittedly hard to go from a standing start to sliding across the dance floor on your knees to 'Livin' on a Prayer', so if people are pestering you to join in – or you want to but feel silly – wait until the floor is heaving, and insert yourself at the edges. Once you start, it's fine; it's getting going that's tricky, so choose a track you love, and move however you want – whether that's a nervy shuffle or a wild air guitar solo. By the second or third song, there'll be no dragging you off the floor.

Big birthdays / big nights out

You may think that this is going to be one of the hardest to cope with sober, but in fact, when you're surrounded by people, music, noise and a giant party, you're going to feel – and indeed be – much less noticeable. Parties and nights at heaving clubs are all about mingling, yelling in people's ears over the music and moving along to speak to someone else, so it's unlikely that many people are going to care if you're on the soft drinks. The issues with Big Nights Out, however, are…

Getting in the spirit

A Big Night Out works thanks to the collective atmosphere of 'a good time'. And the way to generate that fast and furiously is to slosh in as much booze as possible and stand back. Usually that means pre-drinking at home, so that you're already well on the way to Drunksville by the time the cab turns up, and ready to party all night when you arrive. However… for those not drinking, being surrounded by people slamming tequila shots as the Uber waits outside is not always fun. Everyone is engaged in a group activity except you, so how can you feel part of things? And you don't necessarily want to become the Head Hen, shepherding everyone in and out of cabs and negotiating with door staff on your swaying friends' behalf.

So, until you're more used to big nights out without the booze, here are some tips:

Arrive a bit late / cut out the pre-drinking and meet everyone at the venue. (This also gives you time to eat something first, which, let me guess, your friends won't have bothered to do.)

The rising fun / noise / crazy level is infinitely more noticeable when you're sober / suddenly everyone's yelling over everyone else, and all you're thinking is, 'If you all just stopped screaming, you could actually hear each other.' You're on Planet Normal Conversation, they're on Planet Excited Nonsense Shouting. The best solution is, don't talk. Dance. And if there is no dancing…

Be the photographer / nobody remembers to take pictures when they're very drunk. Make sure you do – not only will it be highly entertaining tomorrow, it may also be useful for blackmail further down the line. Joke.

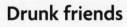

Drunk friends

This is most likely to be an issue on a Big Night Out. Drunk friends can easily become emotional, rambling, sad, aggressive, wandering-off-and-getting-lost friends. As the sober one, you may feel it necessary to look after them, which is fine as long as they're easily poured into a cab, or grateful to be steered away from the idiot at the bar. But drunk people often become boring yet volatile (needy, repetitive, oversensitive), so unless you're actually enjoying their company, reserve the right to leave early. Big parties are tiring – by midnight you may be more than ready for your pumpkin carriage.

FOMO

Fear of Missing Out is one thing – FOMO when you're actually at the event is another. But it can be tough to enjoy yourself when everyone's uninhibitedly having a whale of a time, and you're feeling like you're on the outside looking in. Again, it's a matter of adjusting your expectations. Go to the party / night out intending to see your friends, enjoy the music and be part of something. Don't go expecting a night that gets wilder and more fun as it wears on. When you're sober, the usual 'fun' trajectory flips – the most enjoyable part of a night is usually at the beginning. Assume that's the case and you won't be quite so disappointed that you're not the one trying to scale a lamp post with a kebab on your head at 1am.

Office parties

It's true that drinking has historically been the only way to get through the nightmare of an office Christmas party or bonding weekend. But a sober office get-together requires a different kind of approach. Rather than simply drowning out the white noise of colleagues and their weird lives with booze, this time, decide to find out something interesting about each one of them. Here are a few handy questions to have up your sleeve:

/ **What's your favourite food?**
/ **What's your desert island film?**
/ **What's your favourite cartoon?**
/ **Have you ever seen a ghost?**
/ **If you could travel to any historical period, what would it be?**
/ **Dogs or cats?**

These are useful ways to cut through the usual hellish chat about commuting and the ongoing building work on Level 3, and find out something real about the people you spend most of your waking life with.

Failing that, think of yourself as an anthropologist, studying the strange rituals of 21st-century office culture and alcohol. Embracing any detachment you feel makes it far more enjoyable than trying to fight it. A word of warning, however – don't tell anyone you're doing this.

Worst-case scenario: you'll be bored senseless, but it won't kill you. And if your boss notices your sobriety, it really can't hurt your prospects. Unless you are the boss, in which case you're very much allowed to leave early.

Christmas and New Year

Is it really Christmas without Baileys, mulled wine, rum punch, eggnog, brandy-spiked hot chocolate, red wine by the fire, Bucks Fizz with breakfast, champagne with lunch, a whisky with the big film? And how can it possibly be New Year without cocktails and champagne at midnight?

Well yes, these things CAN be successfully celebrated without alcohol. While culturally we've come to strongly associate it with drinking, the holiday season is fun in its own right.

Christmas without drink

Christmas is usually spent with family or friends – and while some people understandably drink to take the edge off the brother-in-law, or to blur the misery of the kids being with your ex-husband all day, most of us do it just because we can, and it's expected.

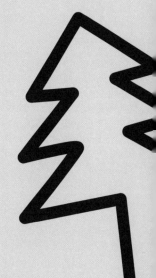

You may well have a family tradition of Bucks Fizz with breakfast on Christmas Day – but does your smoked salmon taste any worse with sparkling elderflower, or a celebratory mocktail? Nope.

And Christmas lunch is so much about the food, it hardly matters what you drink. So the trick of a sober Christmas Day is focusing on what you're doing, not what you're drinking. You're not missing out if others are drinking wine – you're experiencing every moment as it really is, with the excitement of presents, happy kids and silly jokes.

And when it goes wrong, as it inevitably does (an old relative says something racist, a kid has a tantrum), it may be natural to think, 'OK, time to drink through it', but you're not going to. So here's what you can do instead on Christmas Day when you're claustrophobically surrounded by family, and the urge to drink strikes.

Go outside / really. Breathe some air alone for a few minutes. You'll feel better.

Go on Twitter / the campaign #joinin, for people who are alone at Christmas, gathers together tons of kindness and positivity every Christmas Day. It will also make you feel grateful that you're not lonely.

Do something nice for someone / I know, I know, but it helps. Clean up, wash up, help your irritating nephew put his monster truck together. It's a distraction, and it's a bit of moral uplift at the same time.

Have some fake booze / Christmas is a time when 'faux' alcohol really comes into its own. If you're missing the taste and feel of a glass in your hand, pour yourself some Nosecco, or 0.5% ABV wine, and join the others. Sometimes, you have to fake it to make it.

As for New Year...

If you can, take some fake prosecco or champagne along with you and join in with the cork-popping. If you're out, however, and they don't serve it, use the midnight celebrations as a moment to congratulate yourself. Whatever you're drinking, hold it up in a silent toast and say (inwardly, at least), 'I've done it. I've started a new year sober!'

And if that feels good, imagine how great it's going to feel to start New Year's Day *sans* hangover. It may be tough – but once you've done NYE sober, you can do anything sober.

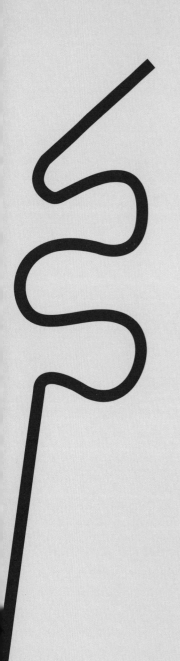

Vacations

This is generally less of a problem if you're on a sunny break with the kids. You may fancy a glass of something cold once they're in bed, but a glass of chilled non-alcoholic beer or a fruity mocktail should do the trick. You're already relaxed; you don't need the extra hit of alcohol to calm you down.

Where it can be tricky is on a group getaway – whether that's boys boys boys in the Balearics, or a gaggle of ageing art enthusiasts in Tuscany.

Because for many, part of the vacation experience is enjoying a drink without the pressure of work the next day, and far away from life's stresses – and if you're not joining in with the shots on the strip / gentle touring of wineries, you can end up feeling that you're missing some crucial aspect of 'relaxing'. Plus, your friends may well be piling on the pressure, with a lot of 'But it doesn't count when you're abroad' and 'One shot of Jägermeister won't kill you'. (Or equally, 'Rosemary, you really must try this astonishing Montepulciano, I insist.')

So here's how to manage it...

boys boys boys /
girls girls girls trip

Make a bit of a joke of your not drinking. The more you try to play it down, the more everyone will wave neon-coloured cocktails at you and make it an issue. Get it out in the open before you go, state that you fully intend to have fun and that this way you're not going to end up doing something you regret. (Chorus of everyone: 'That's what vacations are FOR!')

If possible, don't book yourself onto a trip you know will be a sea of alcohol when you've just quit / that's asking for trouble. Can you go away with your BFF instead, on an activity break, a city break, a spa break… any break where getting smashed isn't the main point?

If you can't get out of the group vacay (and you don't want to), know what you'll drink in advance / look up the bars you might go to and check out the local soft drinks. It's far, far easier to say no to alcohol when you have an alternative you can ask for.

Don't preach / your friends may be vomiting a flashing rainbow of spirits every night, but that's their choice. Unless they're at death's door, don't be the party pooper. Go to bed and leave them to it.

Take headphones and a great playlist / there's nothing like trying to sleep in a paper-walled apartment with all your hammered friends crashing about at 4am.

The civilised drinking trip

It may be civilised (i.e., nobody passes out in the loo and accidentally wedges the door shut), but it can still revolve around drinks on the terrace, wine with lunch, a tour of the vineyard, sunset cocktails, more wine with dinner… Nobody's going to be shouting 'chug, chug, chug' at you, but at the same time, there could be some peevish annoyance at you 'opting out'. Not to mention the bother of splitting the bill when you only had Orangina. So…

Order more expensive food / so that you don't have all the hassle of murmuring, 'But I just had olives and San Pellegrino'. That way, you can focus on fully enjoying the meal, and join in with the bill-splitting equally.

Find 'your' drink / whatever local soft drinks are popular, try them, pick one and stick to it. Then whoever goes to the bar knows what you want and you won't be umming and ahing while everyone's waiting for the wine.

If you're driving to your getaway destination / bring some mixers and syrups so that you can make your own interesting mocktails for evening drinks (see pages 114–131).

Head off on your own if you need to / you don't have to go round a vineyard or to that 'amazing' cocktails-at-sunset event. Go for a swim, take a walk – if you're finding not drinking challenging, make it as easy as possible for yourself by avoiding moments that you know will trigger cravings.

Funerals

Grief doesn't half make you want a drink, if only to temporarily numb the misery. And a funeral is a big gathering of mutual grief – and mutual drinking. If you're bereaved, getting through such a painful event without blurring the edges may seem impossible. But alcohol is a depressant – and a hangover will not improve anything.

If you really can't bear it, your doctor may be able to prescribe you something slightly numbing, such as Valium, but it's less likely that you'll keep adding to your numbness than with booze. 'Feeling the feelings' as they happen can be horribly painful, but if you crush them under a deluge of drink, they will only come back stronger. Drink tea, be with the people you love and listen to what they're saying – words of love and support will be very important to remember later.

Last word...

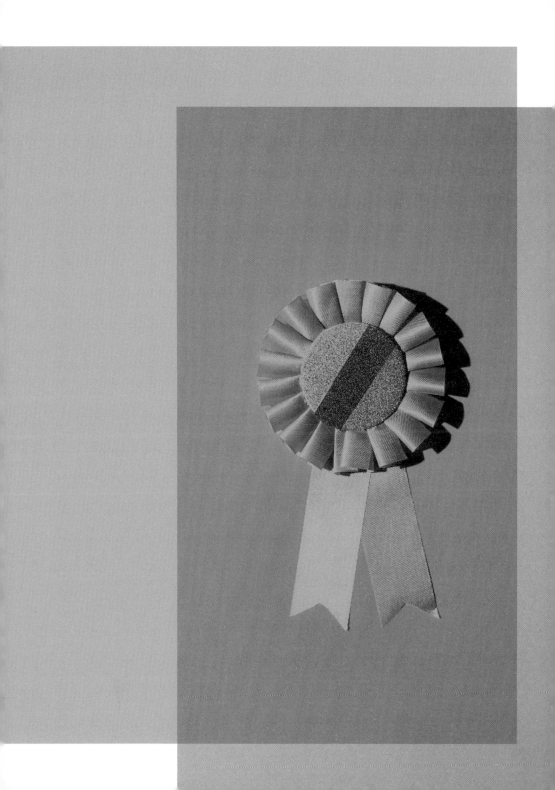

You may not yet be at the stage when it doesn't even occur to you to want a drink. But you will get there. At some point, drinking to get drunk is going to seem a really odd and unnecessary thing to do – like balancing a marble on your nose, or smashing a fairy cake with your fist. You could do it, but why would you? And drinking not to get drunk – again, why bother?

Without alcohol, you will come to appreciate the clarity of knowing whether you actually like someone, rather than simply liking the fact that you're drinking together. You'll love the feeling that you can leave a party whenever you want. (If you're having a great time, though, stay till 4am, fill your boots.) But if you're not, you will recognise that it would be a great idea to leave when you feel like it, rather than sinking another glass to try and prolong the fun you're not really having. You will look afresh at your group of friends and understand, perhaps for the first time since you were 16, that you can choose to hang out only with people who are supportive and fun and good to be around, because it's a lot easier to tell when you're sober. You'll even find that you're only going to bed with people you actually like and fancy. (This is also helpful if you're married to them.)

And of course, you won't wake up with your heart pounding, feeling sick with hangover guilt about what you did and said in the hours you can't remember. (Or sick with a toxic, pounding headache that feels like gnomes are smelting horseshoes in your skull, while a trapped hornet whirrs relentlessly behind your eyes and you can't even escape your own clammy shroud of sweat because your body has been drained of water molecules overnight and you're too weak to move.)

Without drink, you may even find you have more energy. You may lose weight, gain confidence and feel determined to change other things about life for the better too – whether that's leaving a dead-end relationship, having the balls to apply for a new job, travel the world or take to the stage… but let's not get ahead of ourselves.

The main thing for now is that you're cutting down or not drinking alcohol at all. And in one way, that's a tiny thing – it's just deciding to do what's best for you. But in another way it's huge. And life-changing. And you should be really bloody proud of yourself.

L

lime juice
  Cosmopolitan 128
  Mojito 126
limits, alcohol 11
loneliness 76

M

Manhattan 118
Martini, Pornstar 121
measures 89
meeting people 42
mint: Mojito 126
mocktails 112–31
  Cosmopolitan 128
  Cucumberbatch 129
  Dark Invader 124
  Forest Fruits Daiquiri 125
  Manhattan 118
  Mojito 126
  Old Fashioned 122
  Pina Colada 120
  Pornstar Martini 121
  setting up a mocktail cabinet
    116–17
  Virgin Mary 130
Mojito 126
money 9
motivations
  for drinking 17, 18–33
  for giving up alcohol 8–11, 55

N

New Year 148, 149
non-alcoholic drinks 108–10, 112–31
  Cosmopolitan 128
  Cucumberbatch 129
  Dark Invader 124
  Forest Fruits Daiquiri 125
  Manhattan 118

Mojito 126
Old Fashioned 122
Pina Colada 120
Pornstar Martini 121
setting up a mocktail cabinet
  116–17
Virgin Mary 130

O

office parties 147
Old Fashioned 122
out-of-control-drinkers 24, 30

P

passion fruit syrup: Pornstar Martini
  121
Pina Colada 120
pineapple juice
  Dark Invader 124
  Pina Colada 120
Pornstar Martini 121
'pretend booze' 80, 101
prosecco, non-alcoholic: Pornstar
Martini 121

Q

quitting alcohol
  fear of 36–49
  fighting the fear of 48–9
  getting started 54–65
  reasons for 6–13
  tips to help 56–60
quiz, reasons for drinking 18–25

R

raspberries: Forest Fruits Daiquiri
  125
relationships 11, 57, 84–7
  dates 102
  and fear of quitting alcohol 44–5
relaxing without alcohol 40–1
rewards 58

rituals 70
routines, changing 59

S

San Pellegrino Limonata: Dark
Invader 124
sex life 87
Shirley Temple 110
shyness, tackling 142
skin 9
sleep 8, 46–7
sober buddies 59
Sober October 54
soda water with angostura bitters 109
speeches 143
staying in 66–89
support, finding 27

T

teas, herbal 81
tiredness 77
tomato juice: Virgin Mary 130

U

units recommended per week 11

V

vacations 150–2
Virgin Mary 109, 130

W

water, sparkling 110
weddings 140–4
wine, non-alcoholic 110
  Manhattan 118
work
  office parties 147
  work drinks 103
worries 9

Publishing Director Sarah Lavelle
Commissioning Editor Zena Alkayat
Editor Harriet Webster
Art Direction / Design Maeve Bargman
Cover Series Designer Luke Bird
Photographer Kim Lightbody
Props Stylist Rachel Vere
Recipe Writer Flic Everett
Production Director Vincent Smith
Production Controller Nikolaus Ginelli

Published in 2019 by Quadrille,
an imprint of Hardie Grant Publishing

Quadrille
52–54 Southwark Street
London SE1 1UN
quadrille.com

ISBN 978 1 78713 422 5

Printed in China

**This book is not intended
as a substitute for genuine
medical advice. The reader
should consult a medical
professional in matters
relating to his / her health,
particularly with regard to
symptoms of addiction or
alcohol-related illness.**